Nurse 101
A Snarky, Sweary, Hilarious Adult Coloring Book

By Peaceful Mind Adult Coloring Books

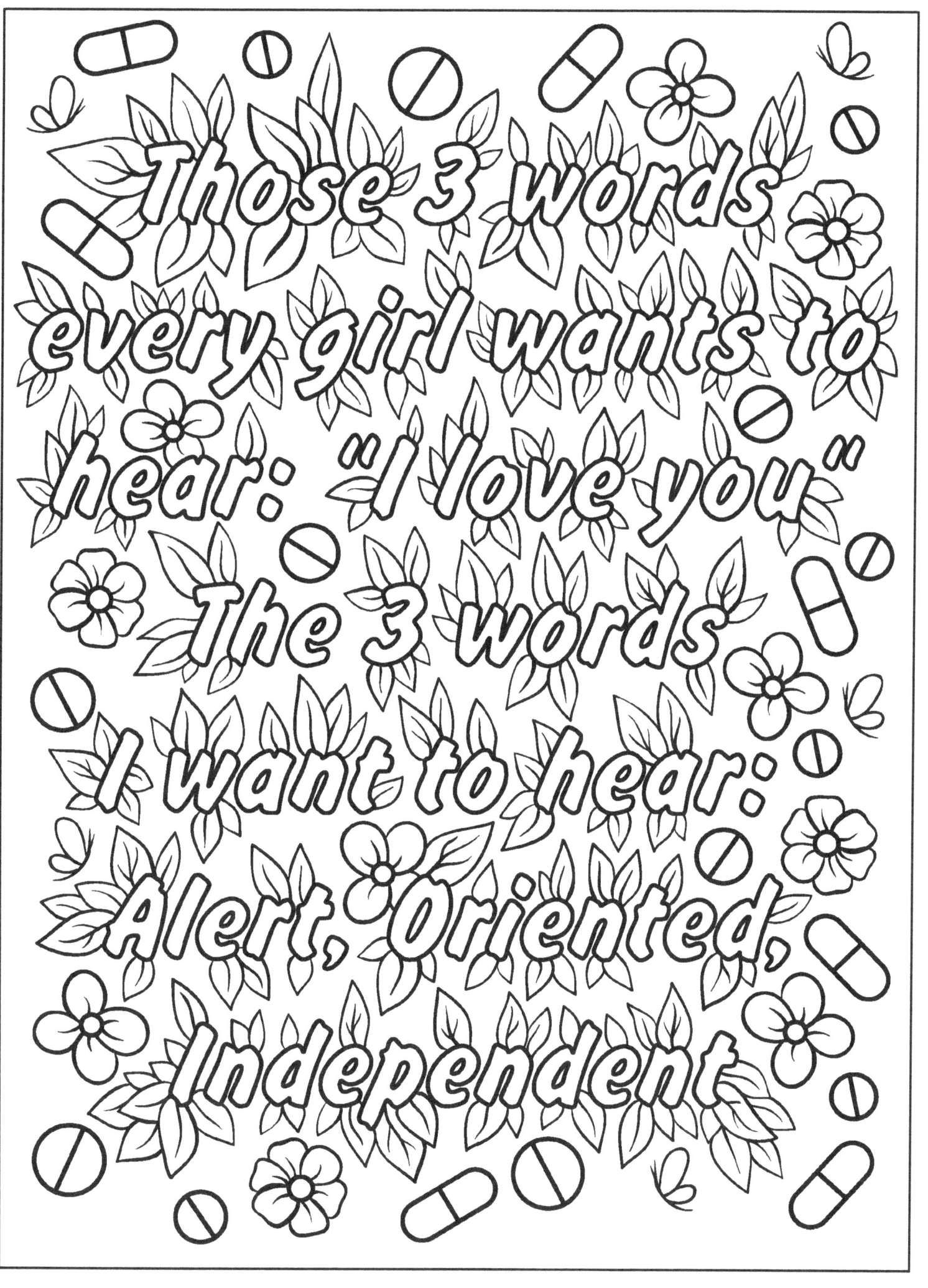

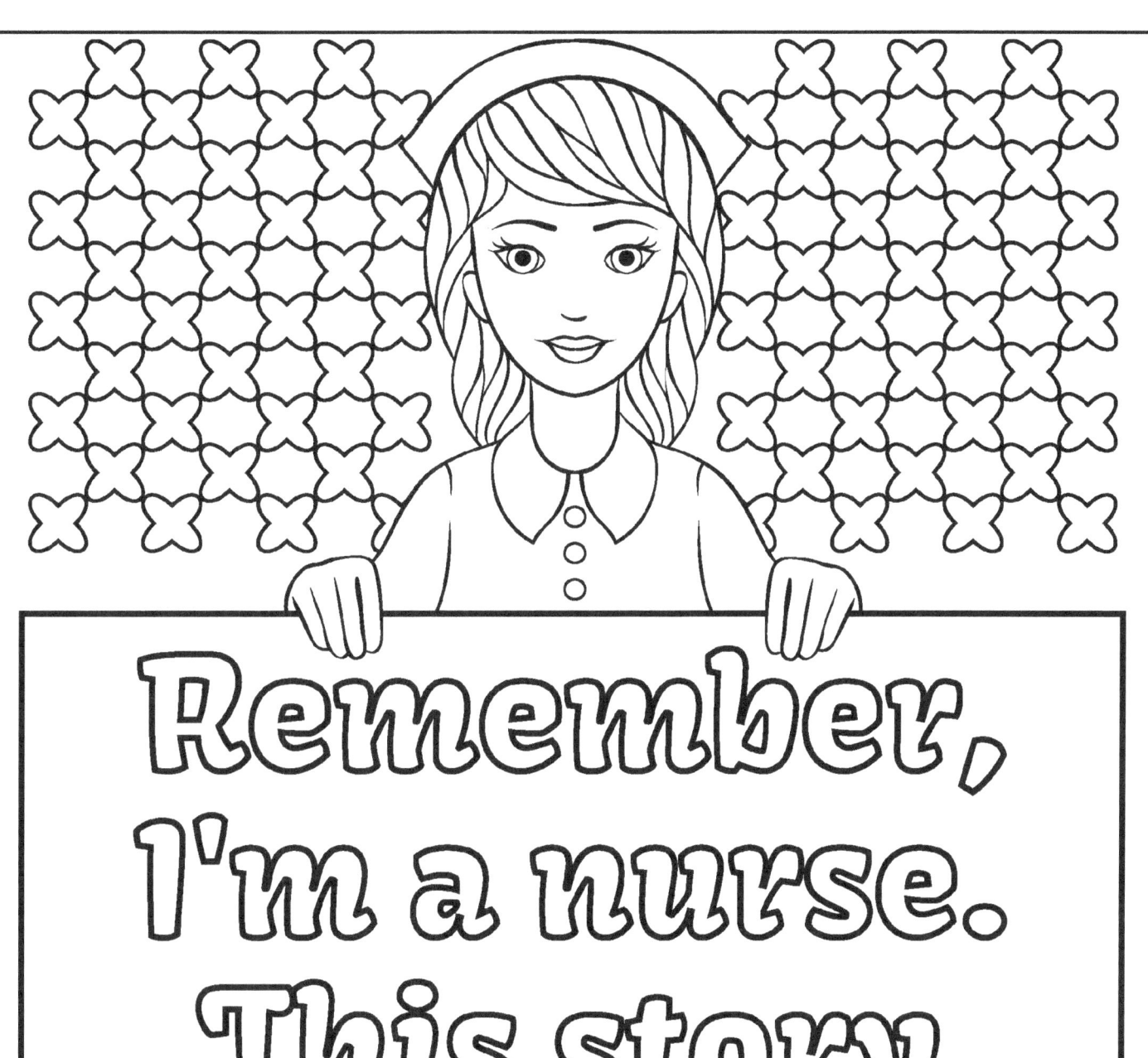

Remember, I'm a nurse. This story needs to be really good to gross me out.

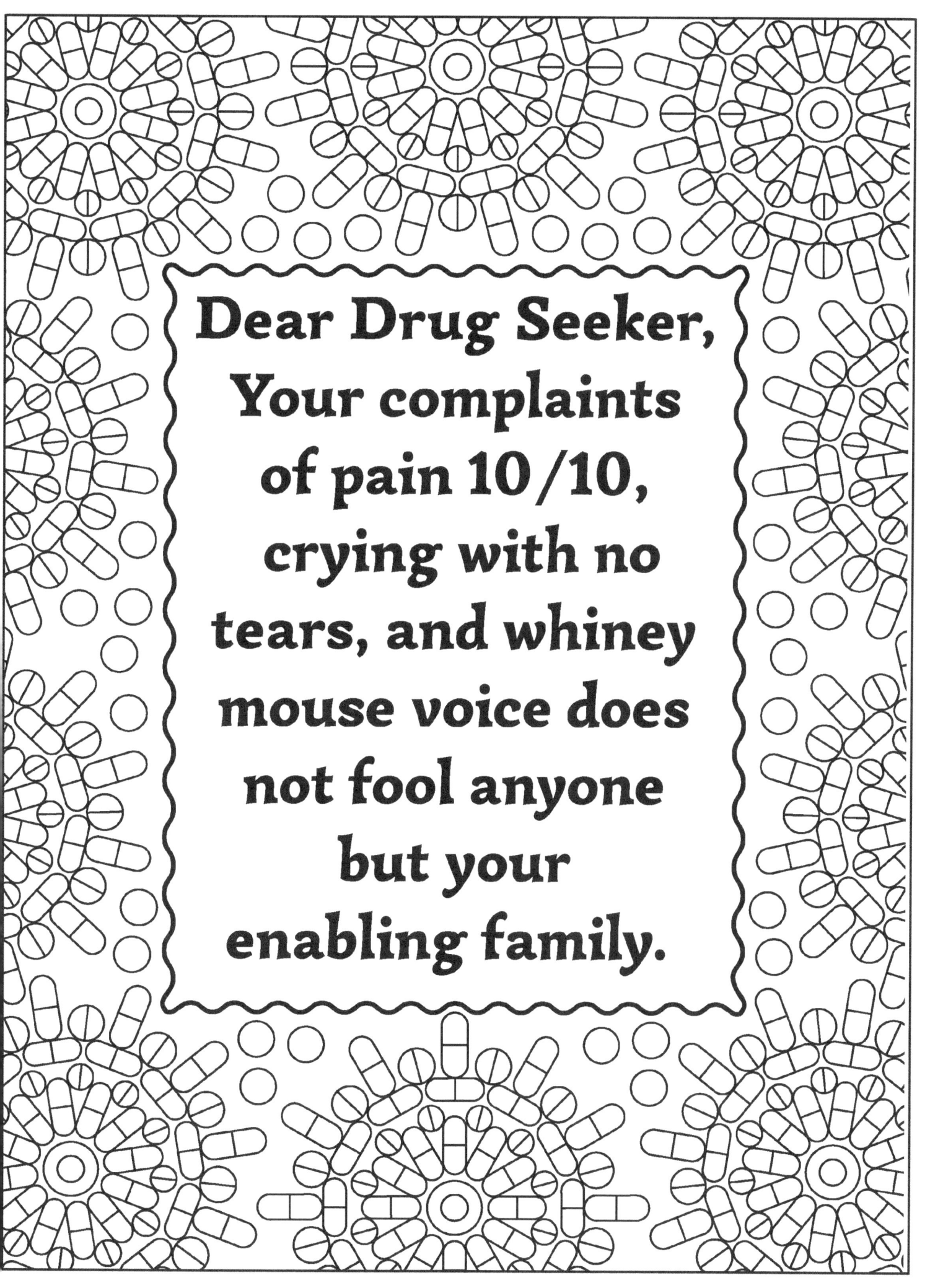

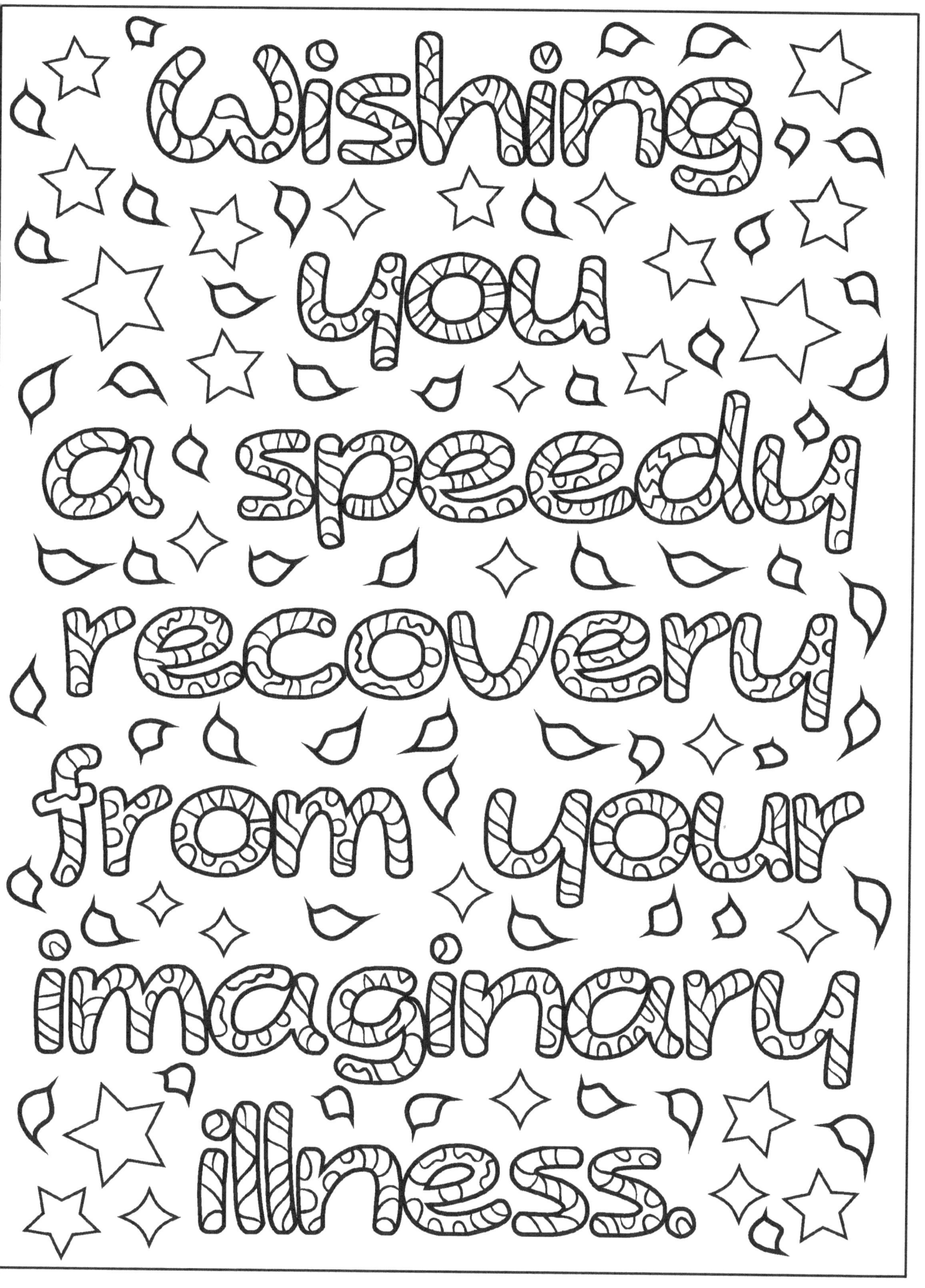

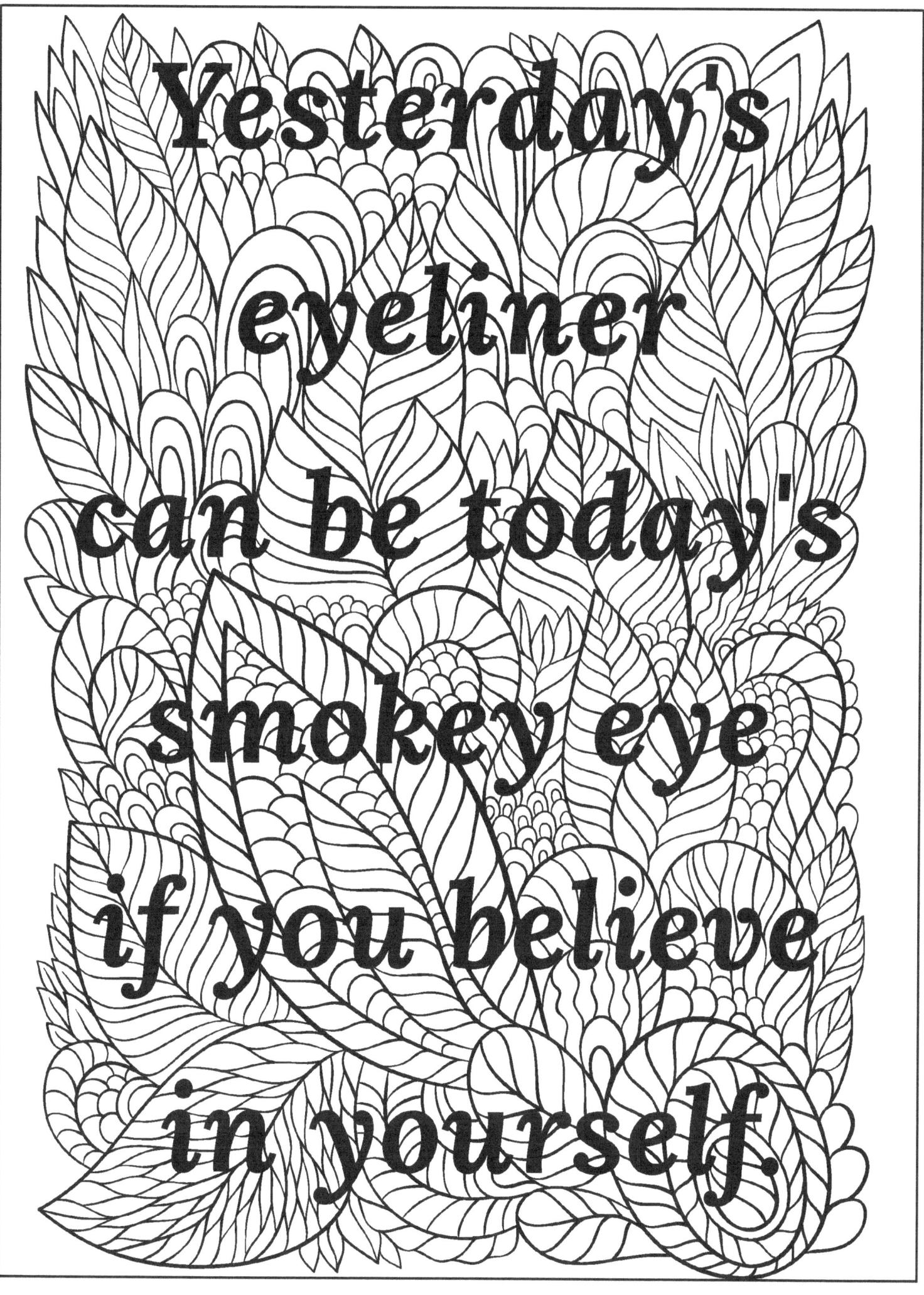

Yesterday's eyeliner can be today's smokey eye if you believe in yourself.

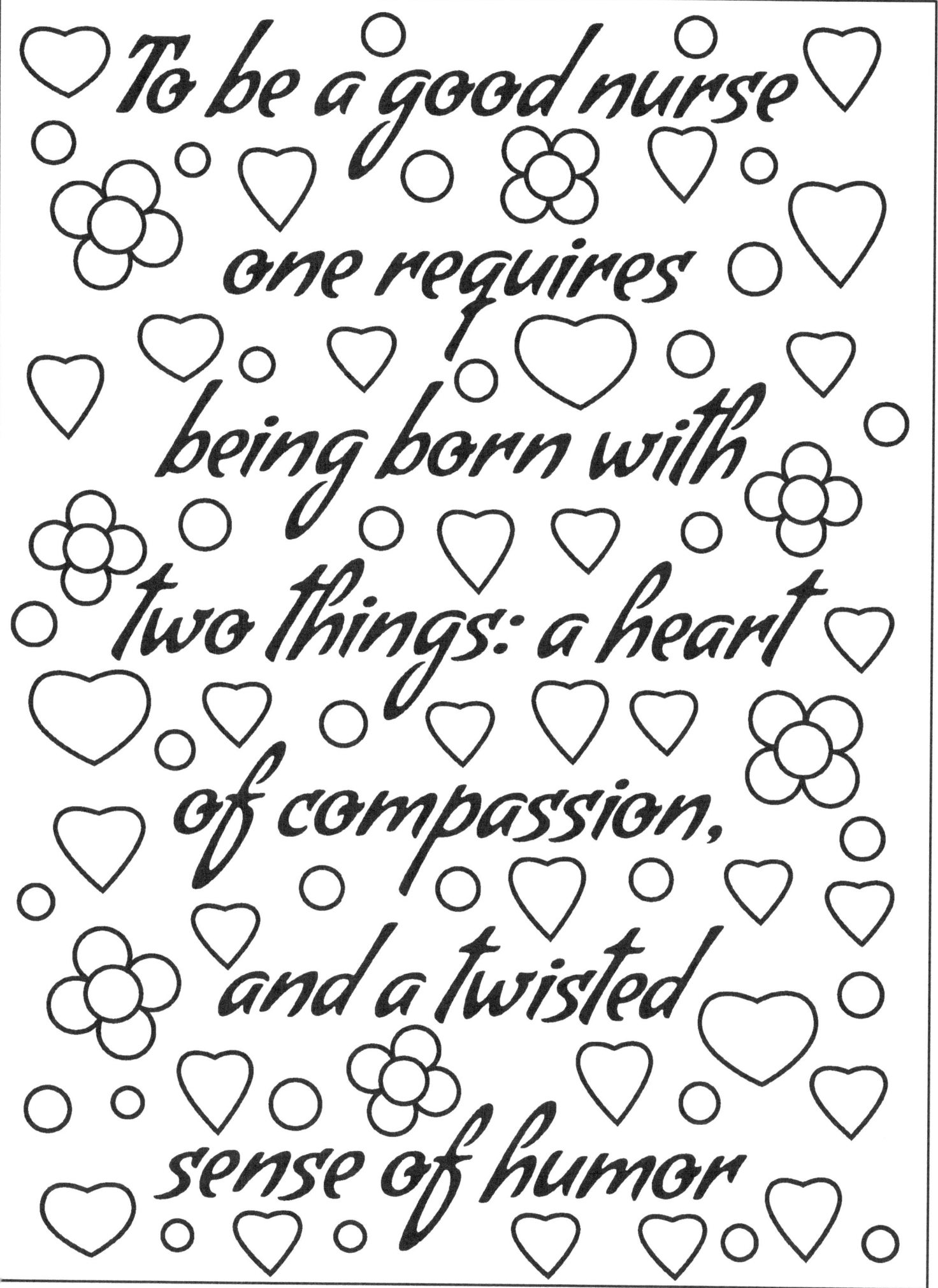

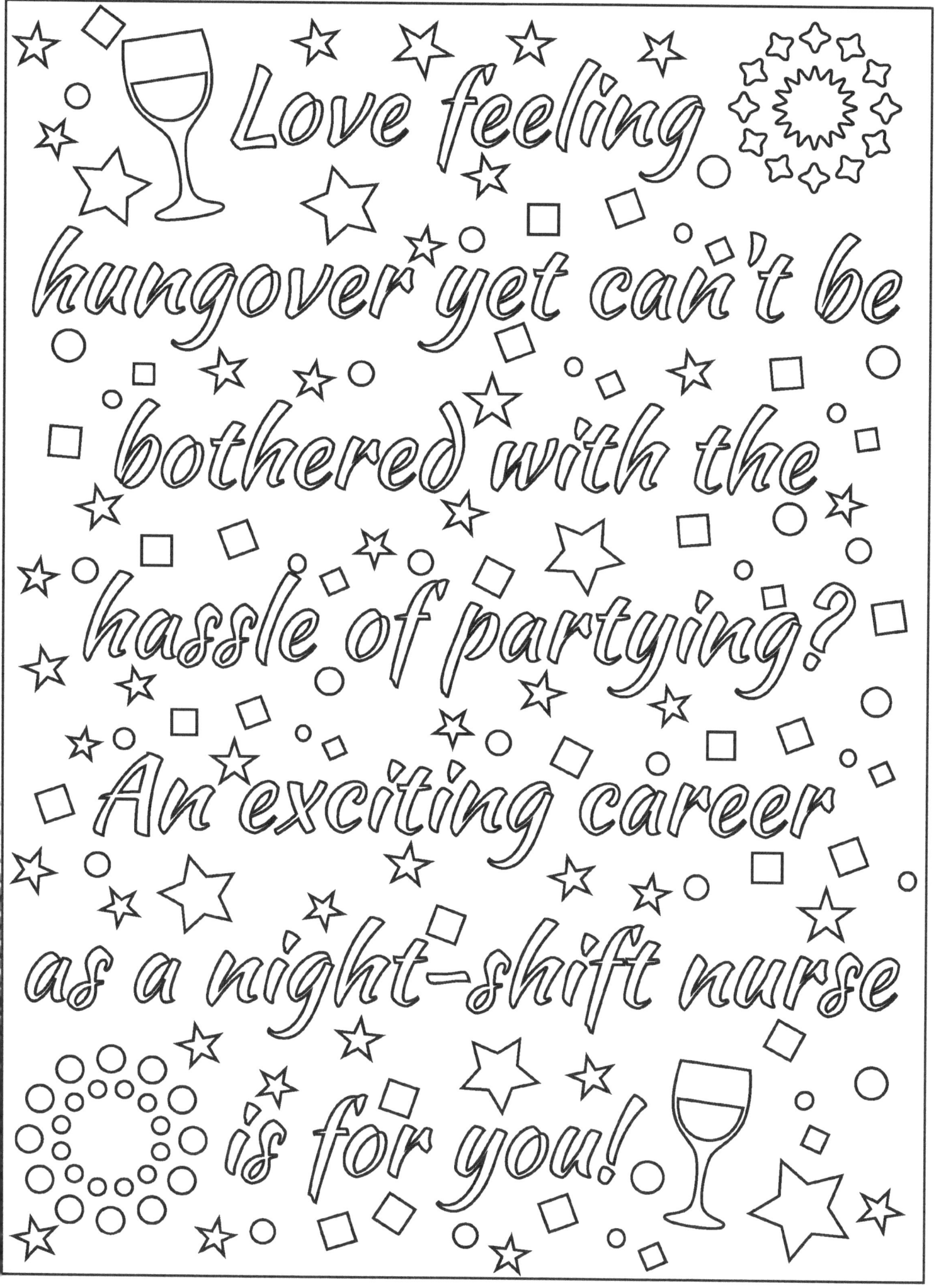

Love feeling hungover yet can't be bothered with the hassle of partying? An exciting career as a night-shift nurse is for you!

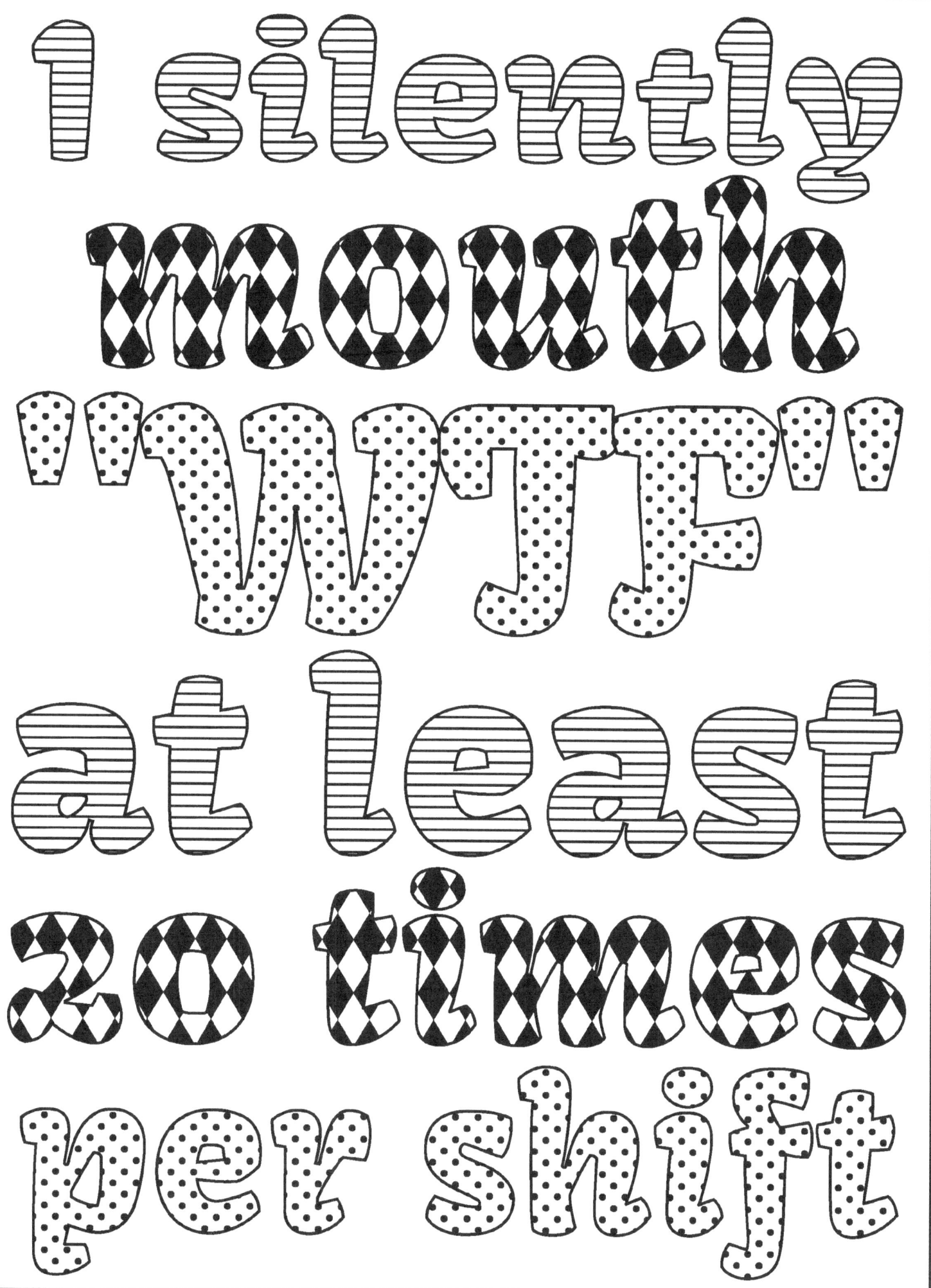

Nursing: A profession where you must also wash your hands BEFORE using the restroom.

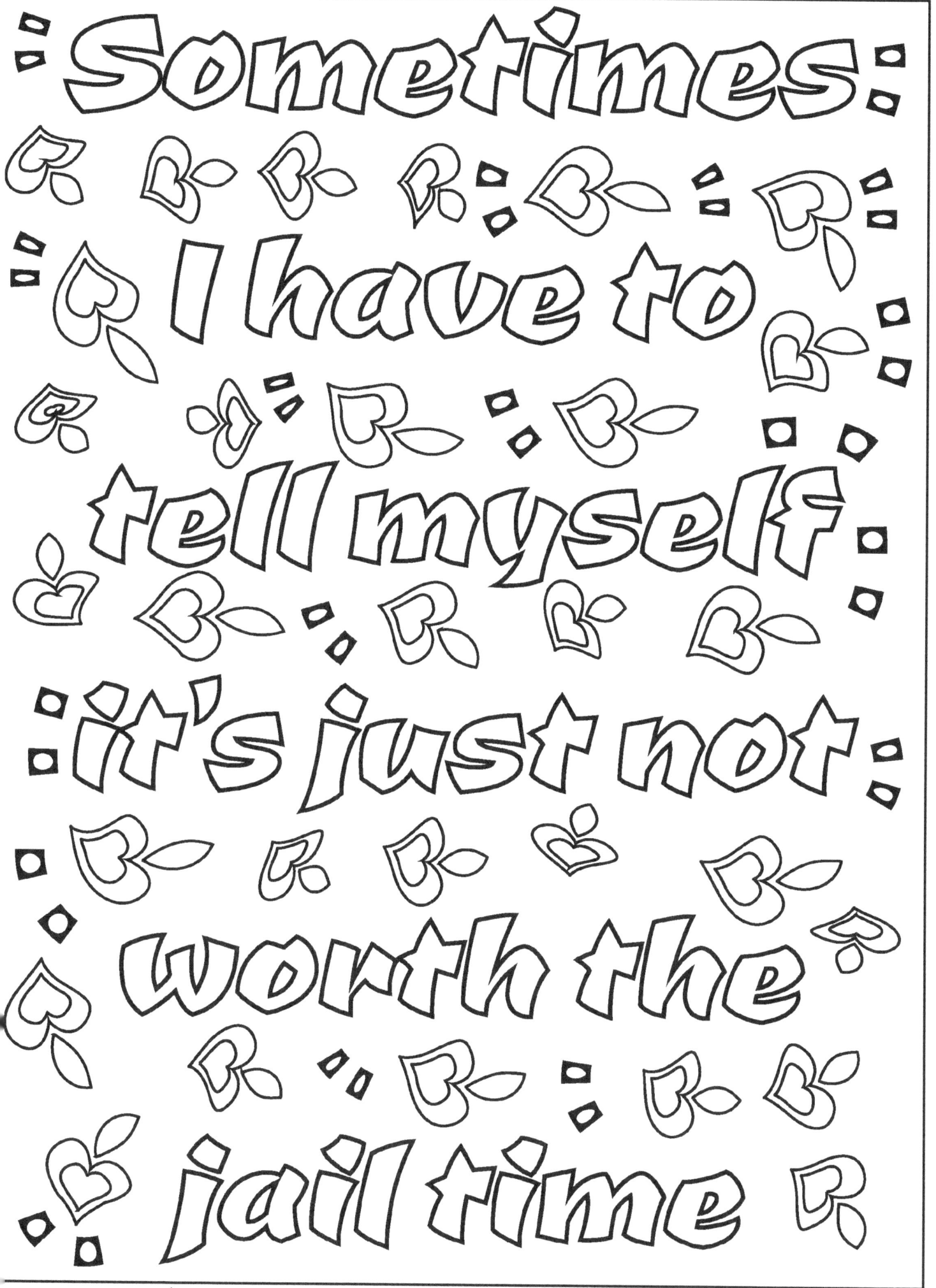

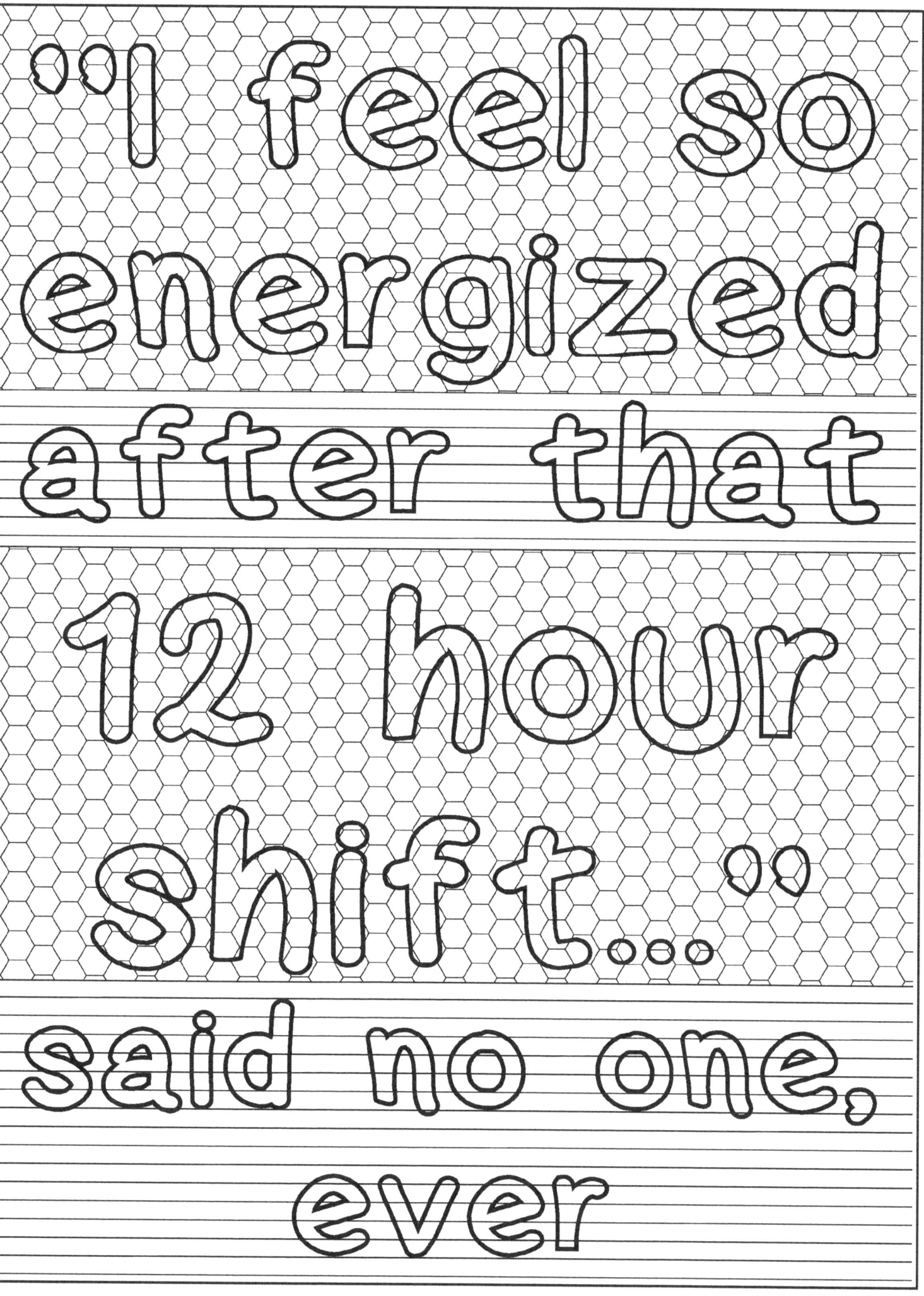

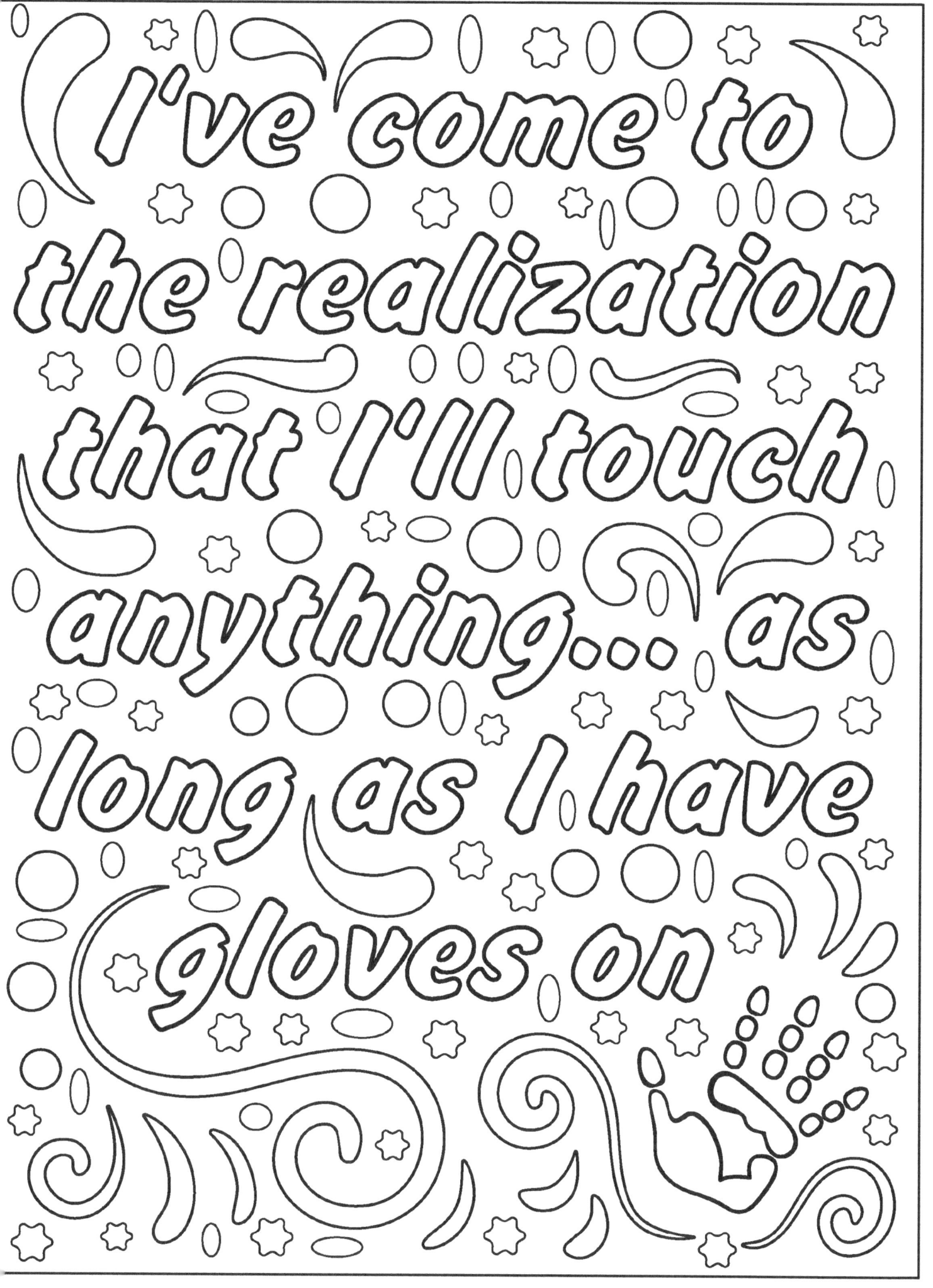

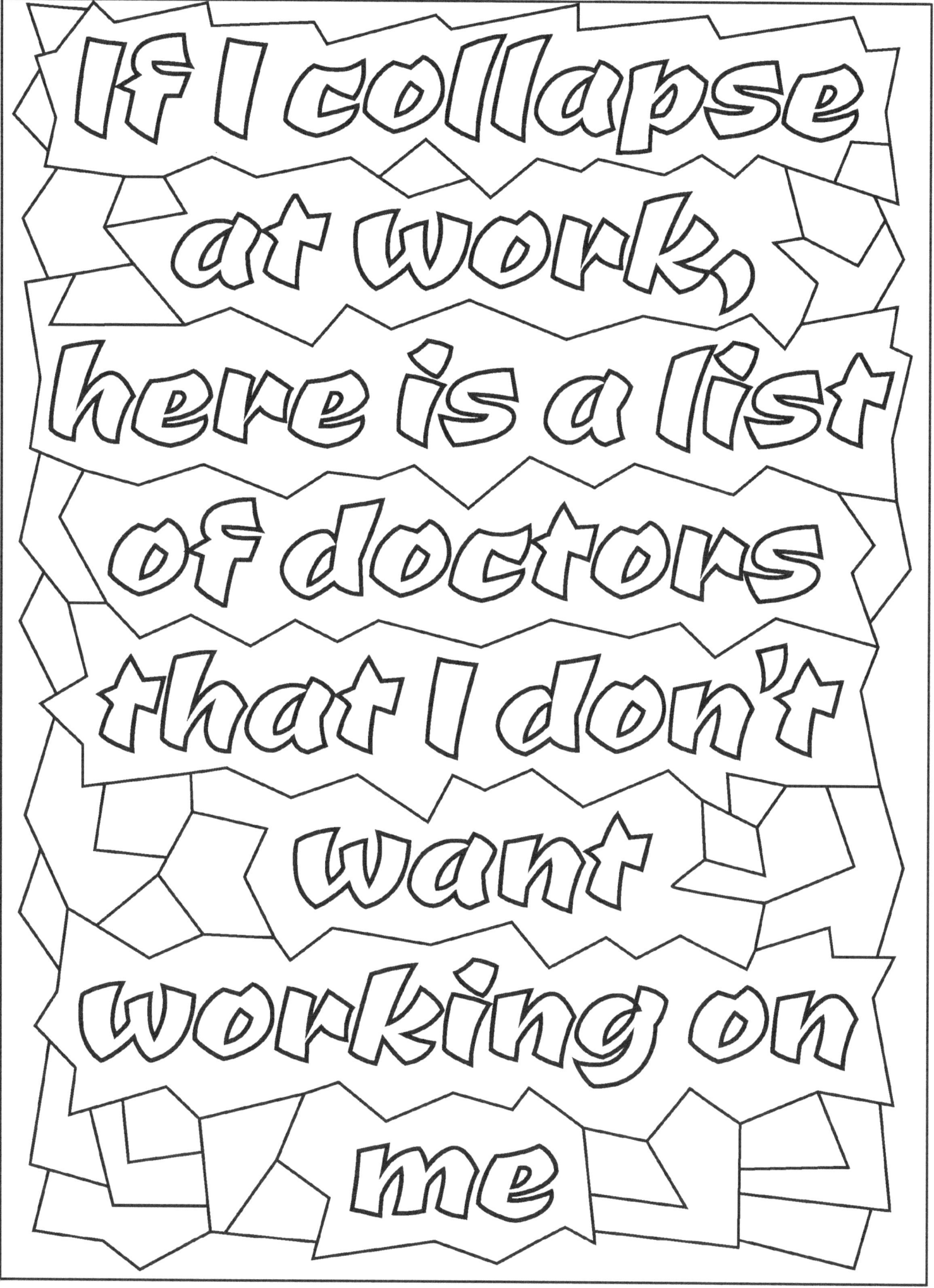

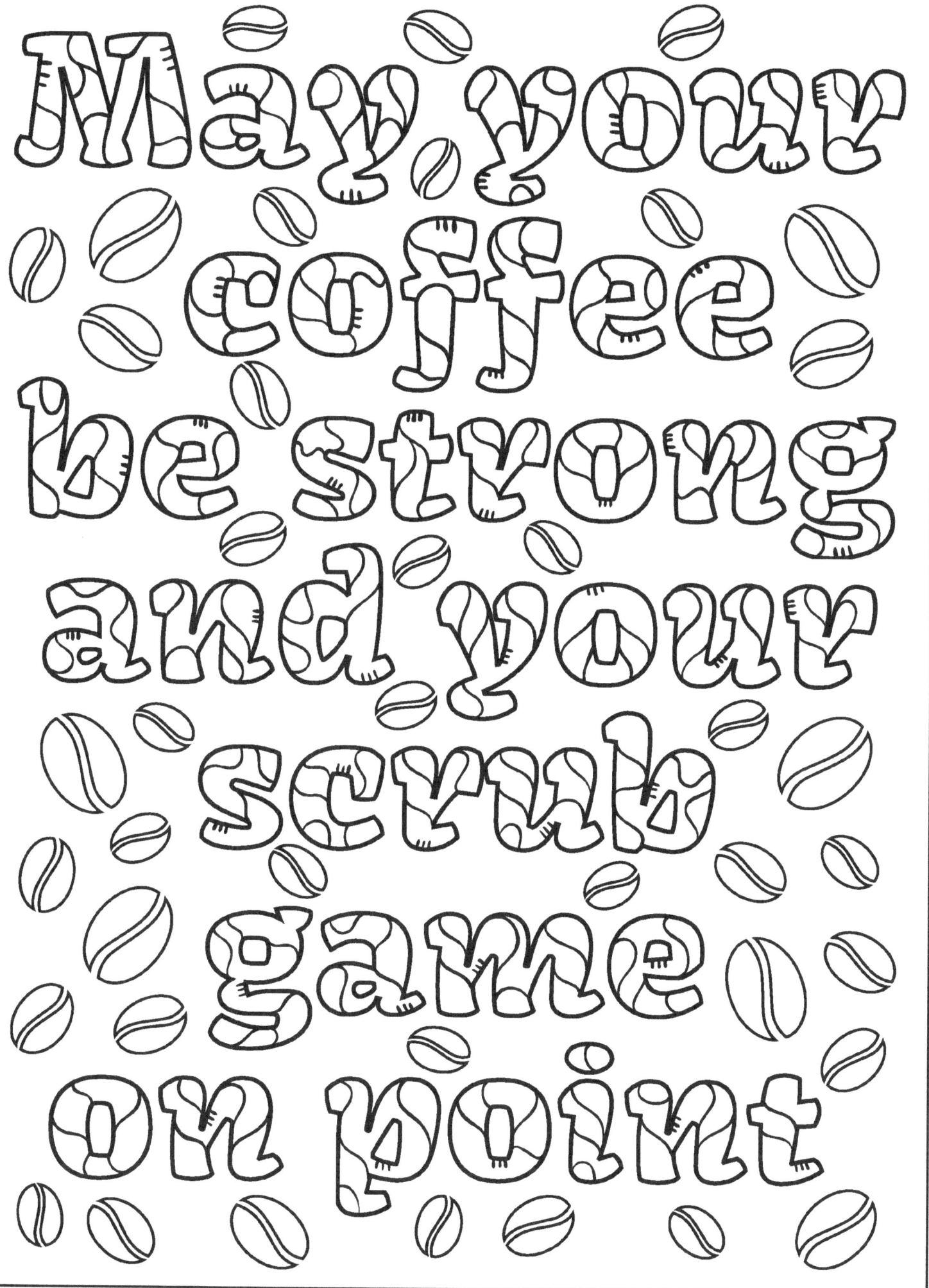

Sure I can do all your work while you sit there and do nothing all day. Why not I have nothing better to do!

NURSE

noun [en·juh·neer]
Someone who does precision guesswork based on unreliable data provided by those of questionable knowledge.
See also: wizard, magician

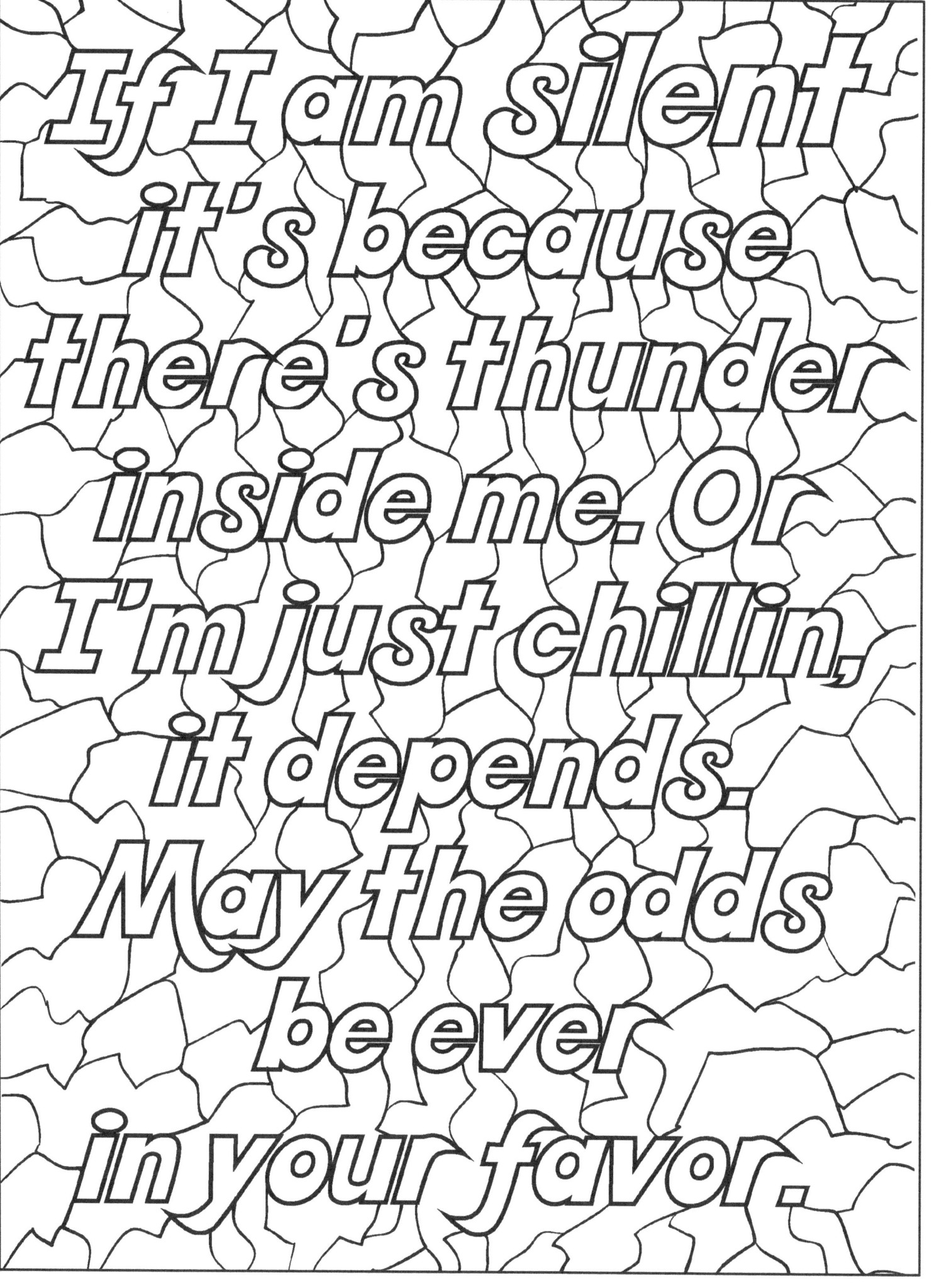

I'm sorry, putting up with your shit isn't on my to do list today.

You think Mondays are bad? Try working weekends, holidays, and 12 hour nights!

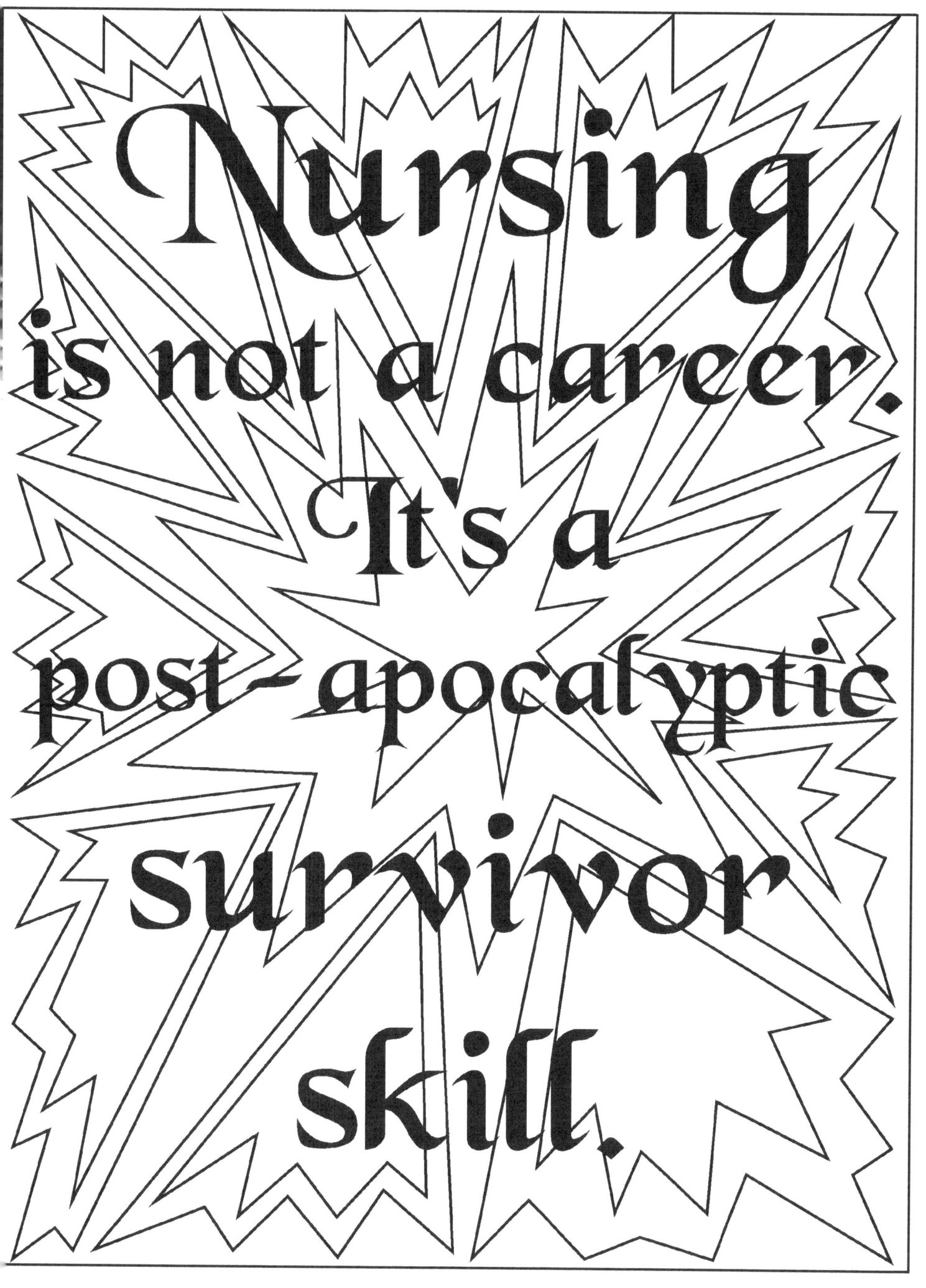

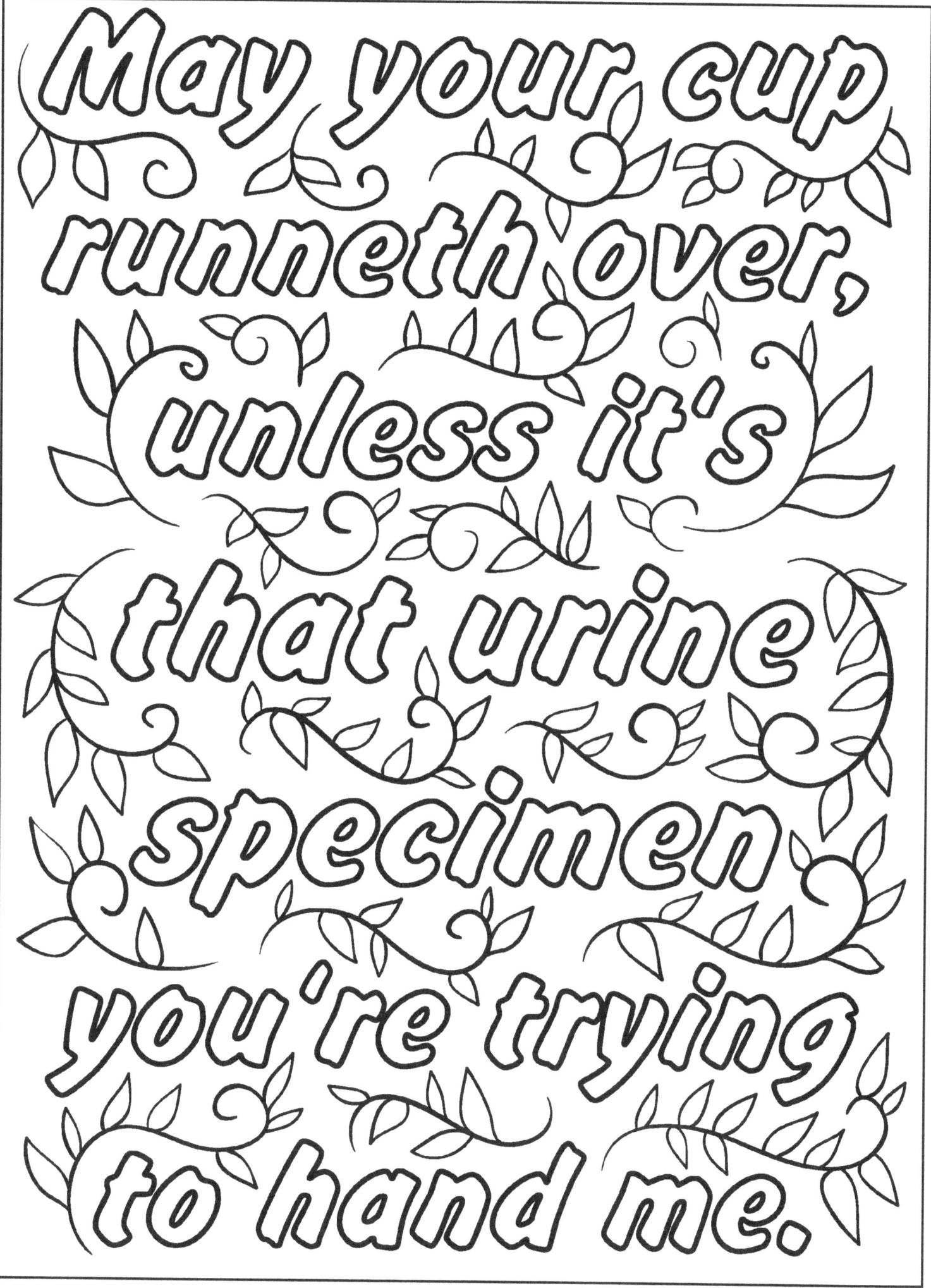

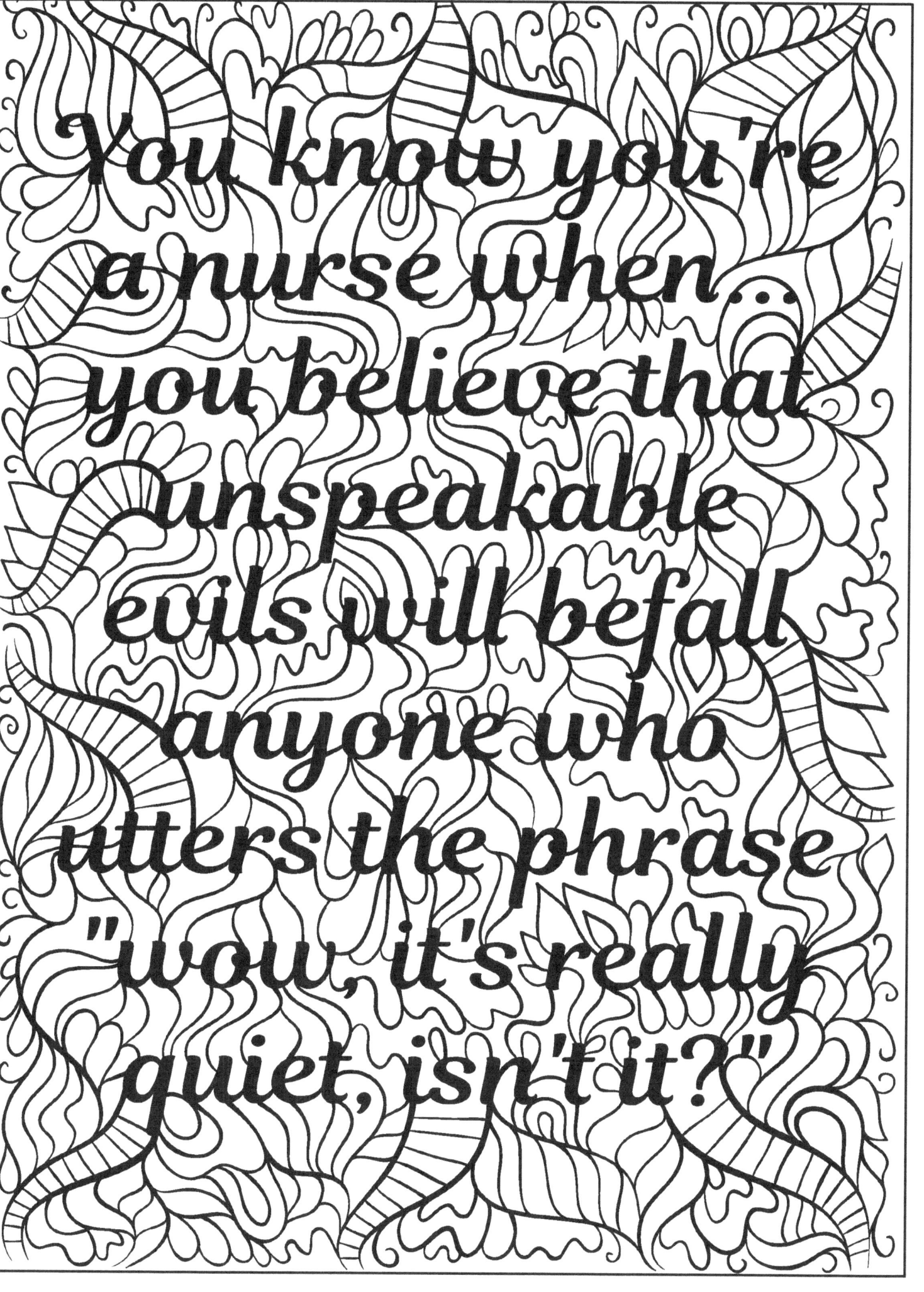

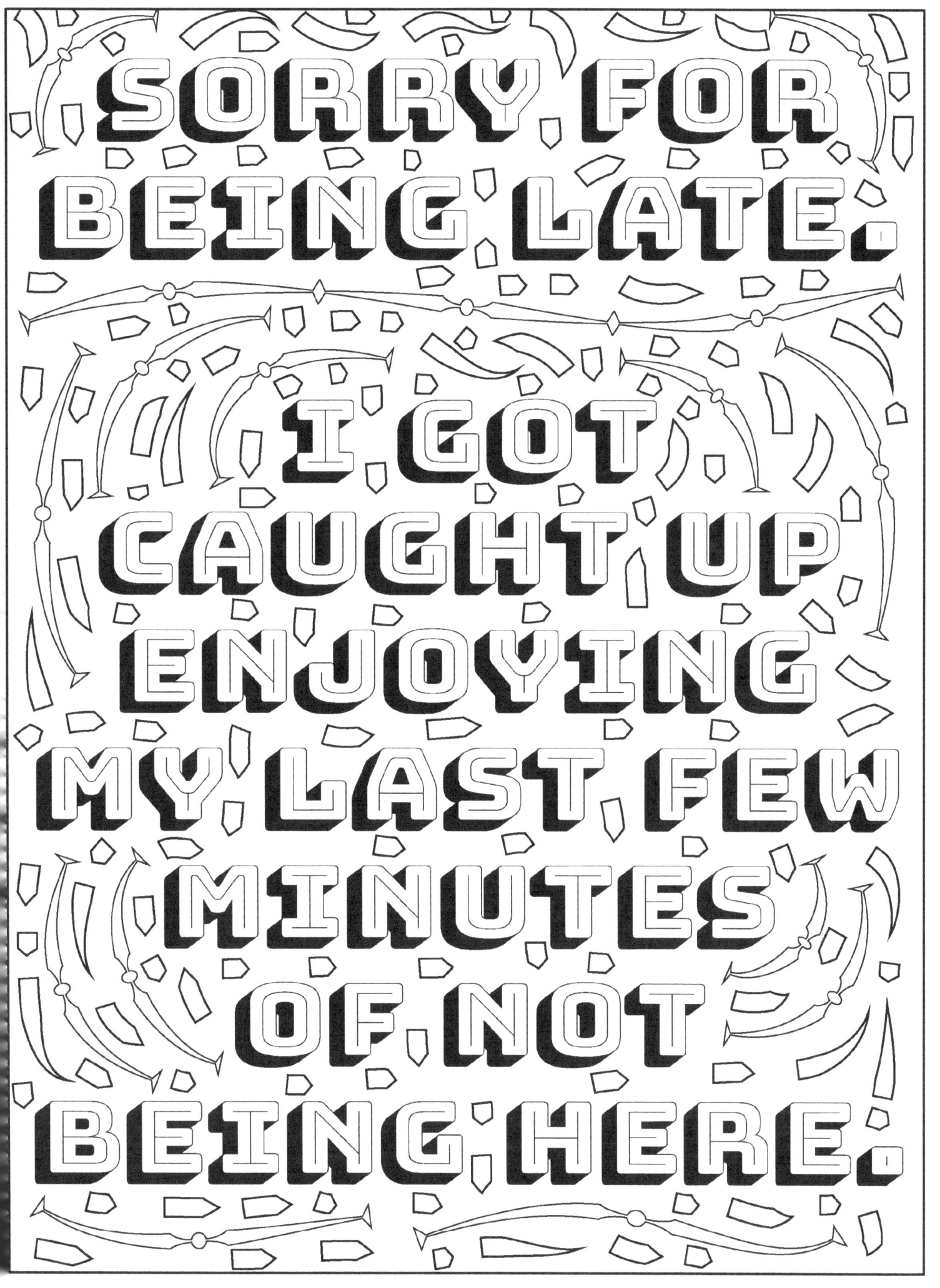

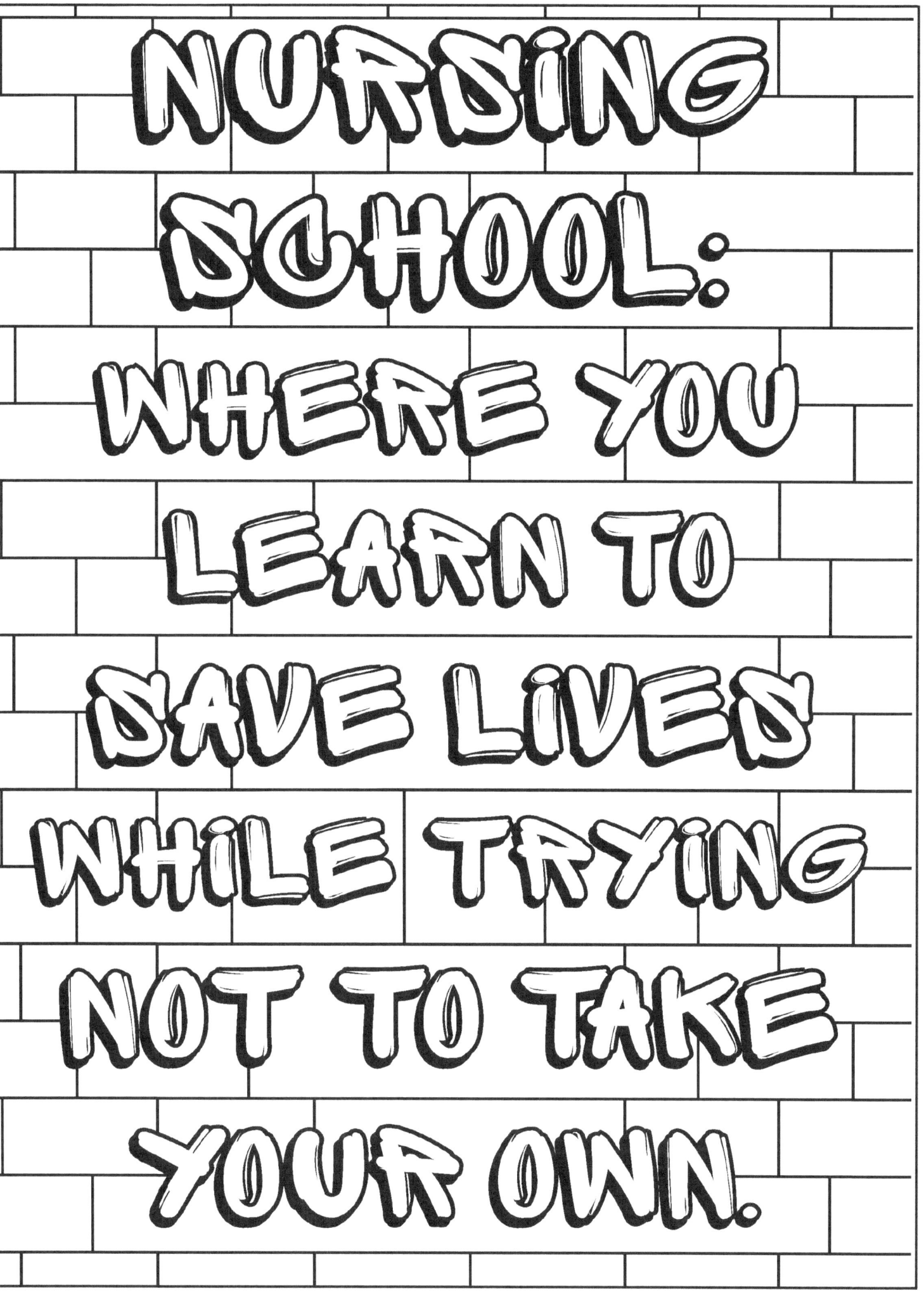

So you need a refill and you don't know what the drug is called? But it's white and round you say???

They say you should walk a mile in someone else's shoes. I'm a nurse, and you'll be walking a hell of a lot further than that.

Please rate your pain on a zero to ten scale. Zero being no pain. Ten being I just force fed you live scorpions and then ripped off both your arms.

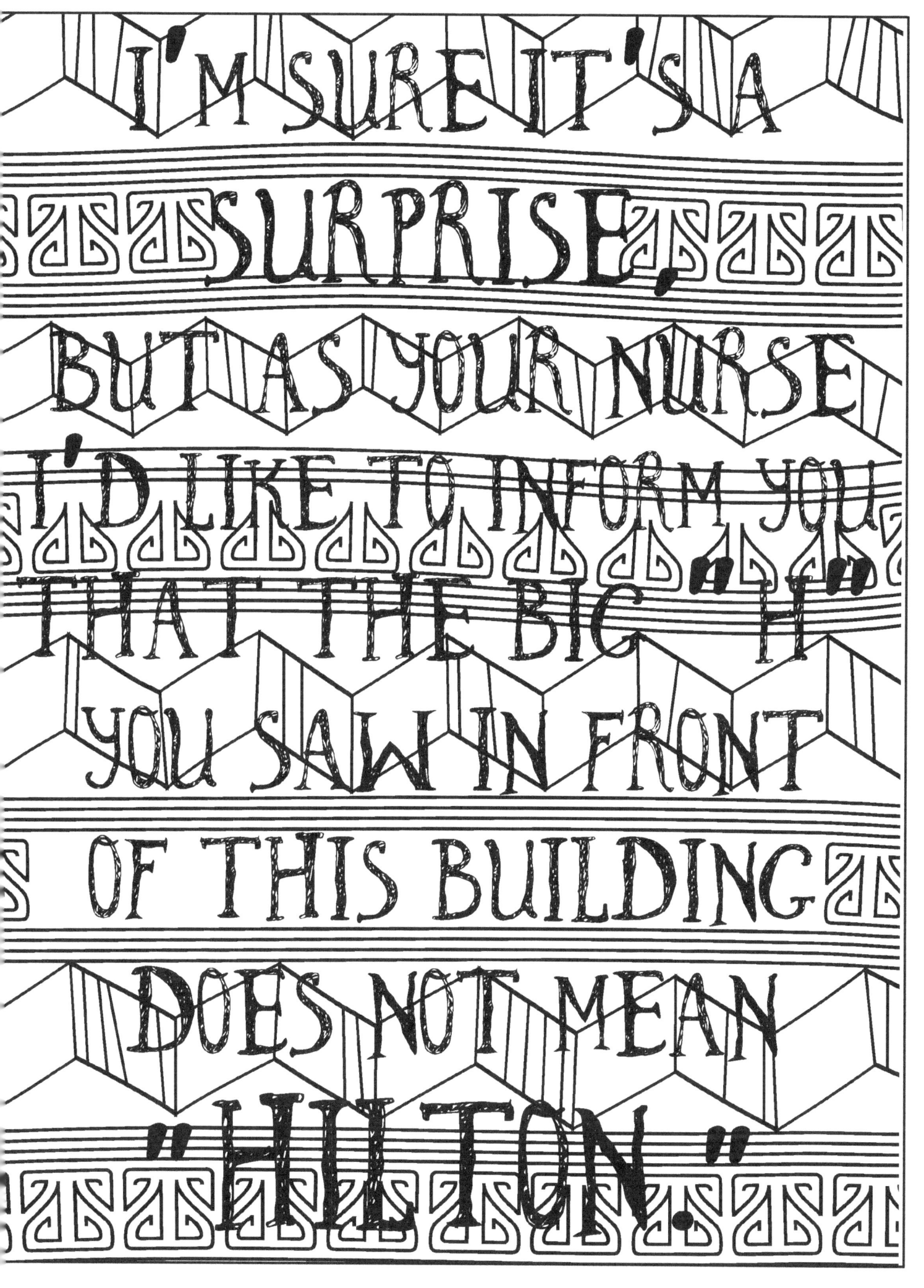

I'M SURE IT'S A SURPRISE, BUT AS YOUR NURSE I'D LIKE TO INFORM YOU THAT THE BIG "H" YOU SAW IN FRONT OF THIS BUILDING DOES NOT MEAN "HILTON."

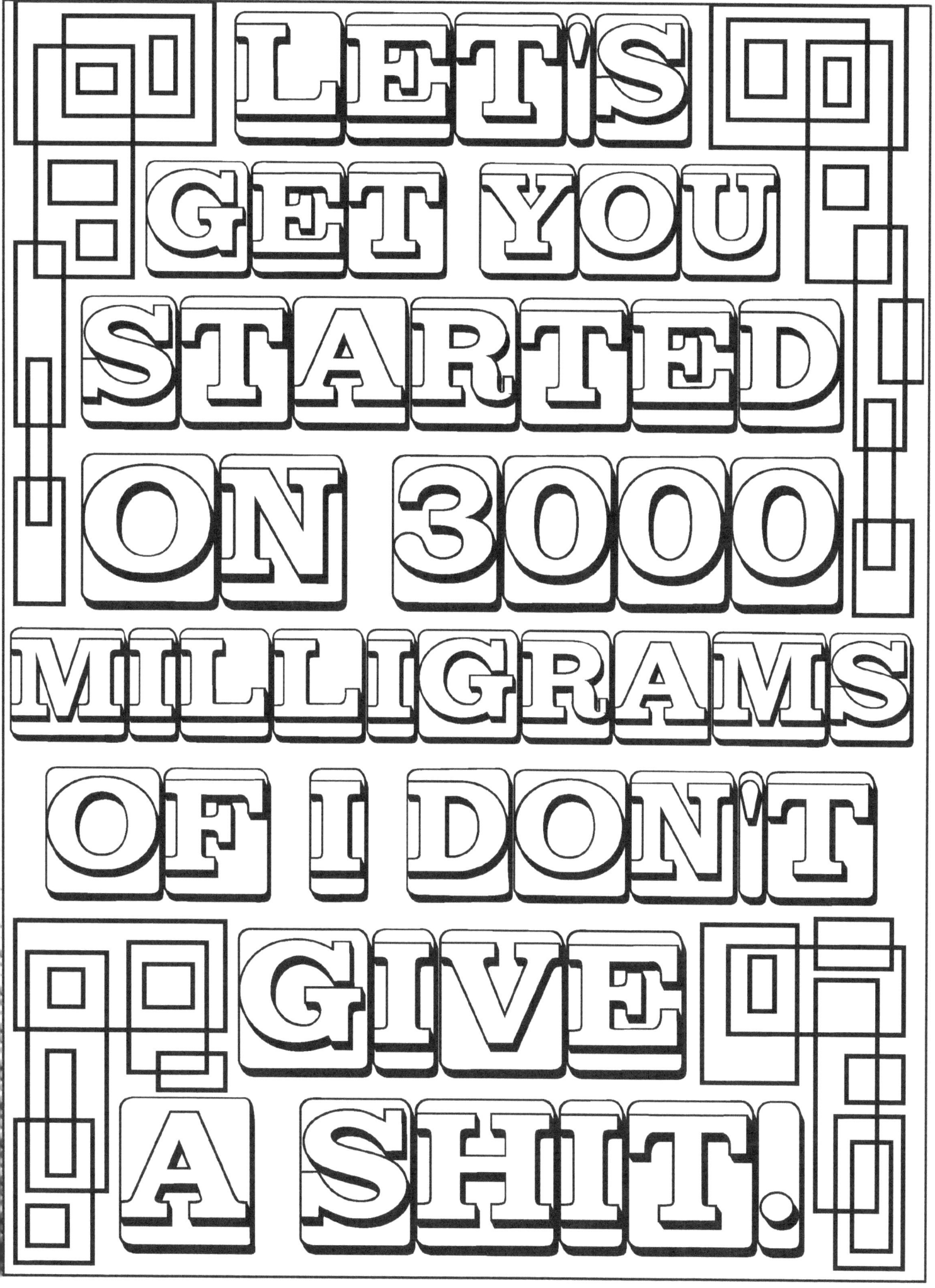

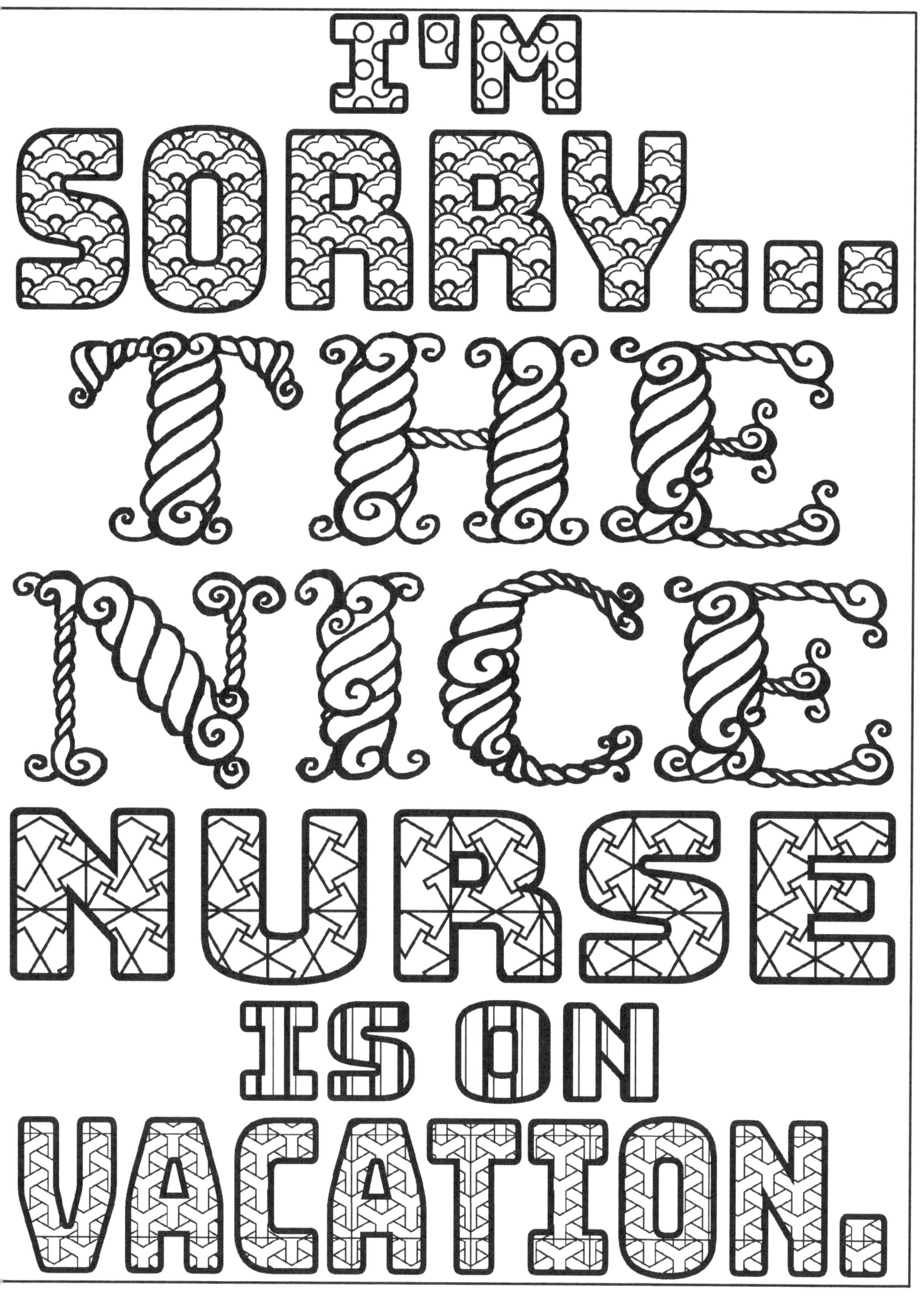

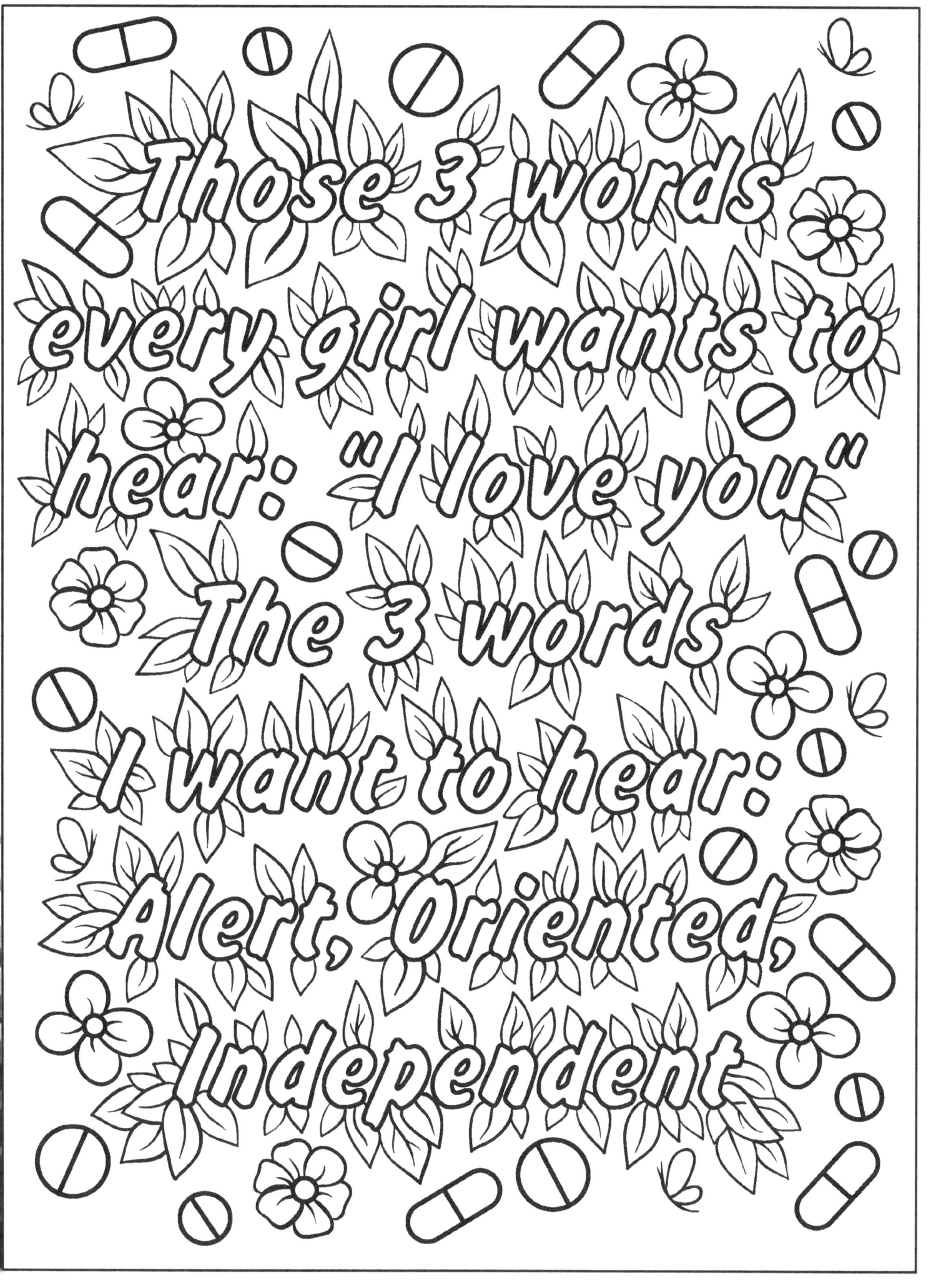

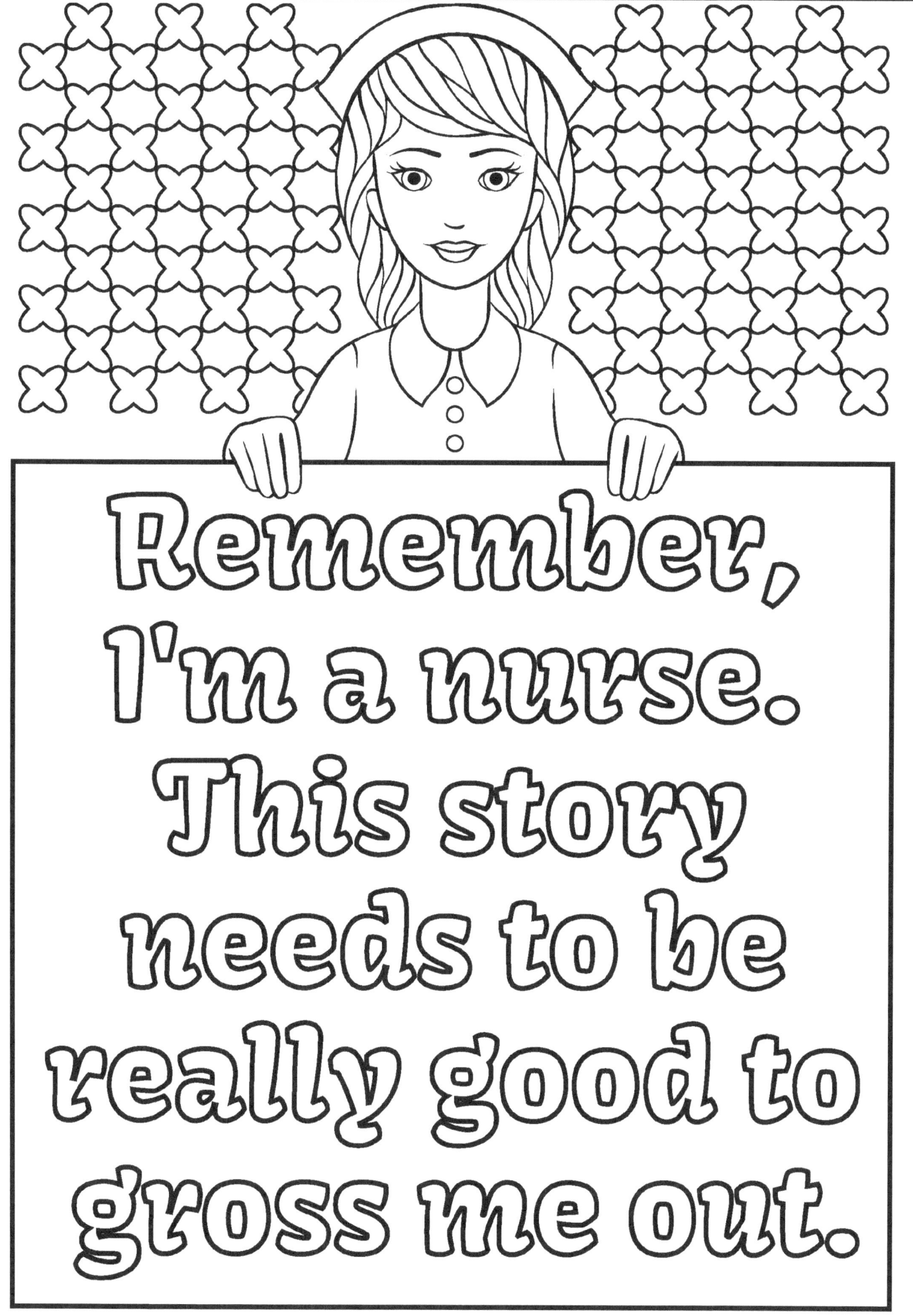

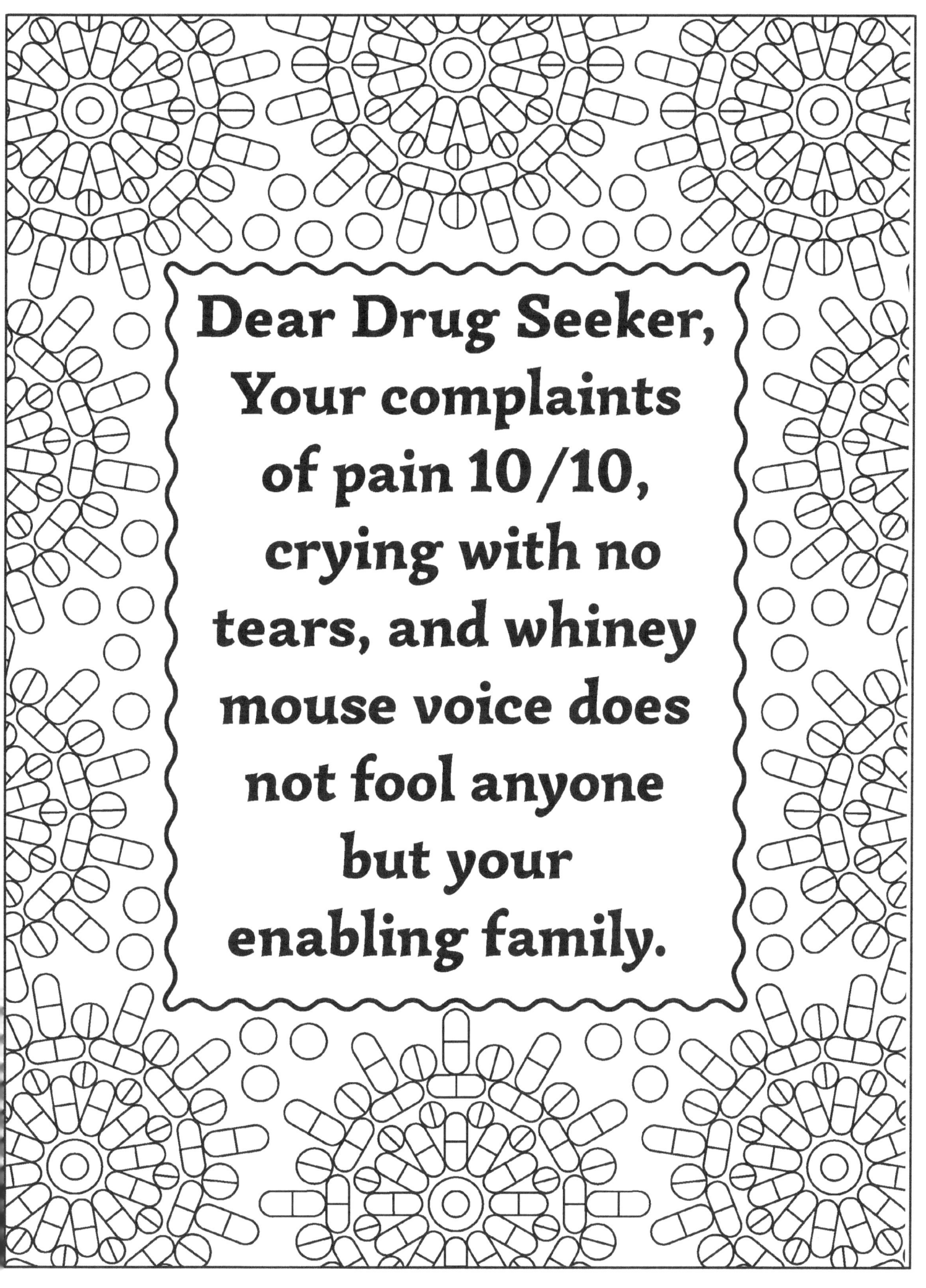

Dear Drug Seeker, Your complaints of pain 10/10, crying with no tears, and whiney mouse voice does not fool anyone but your enabling family.

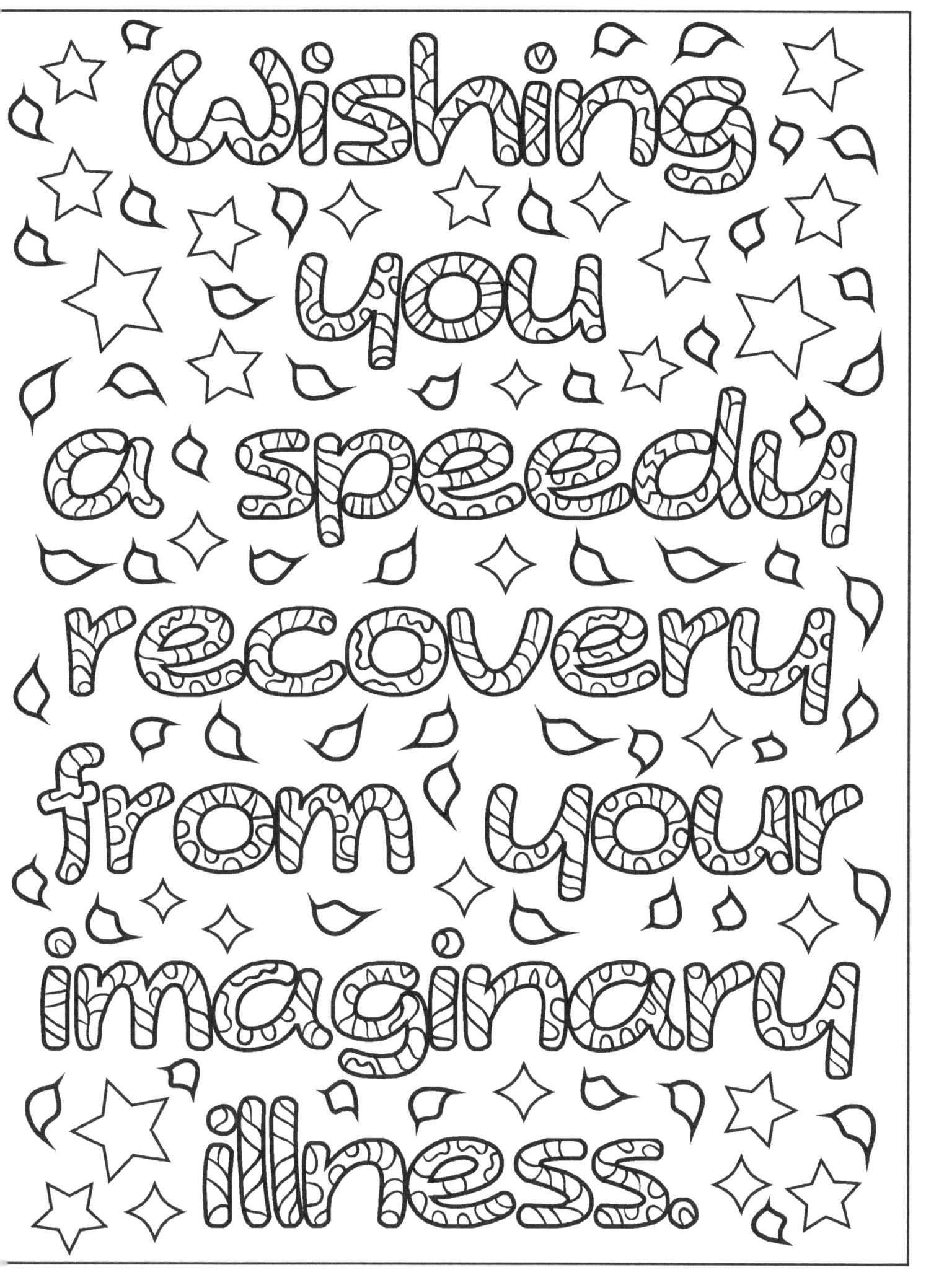

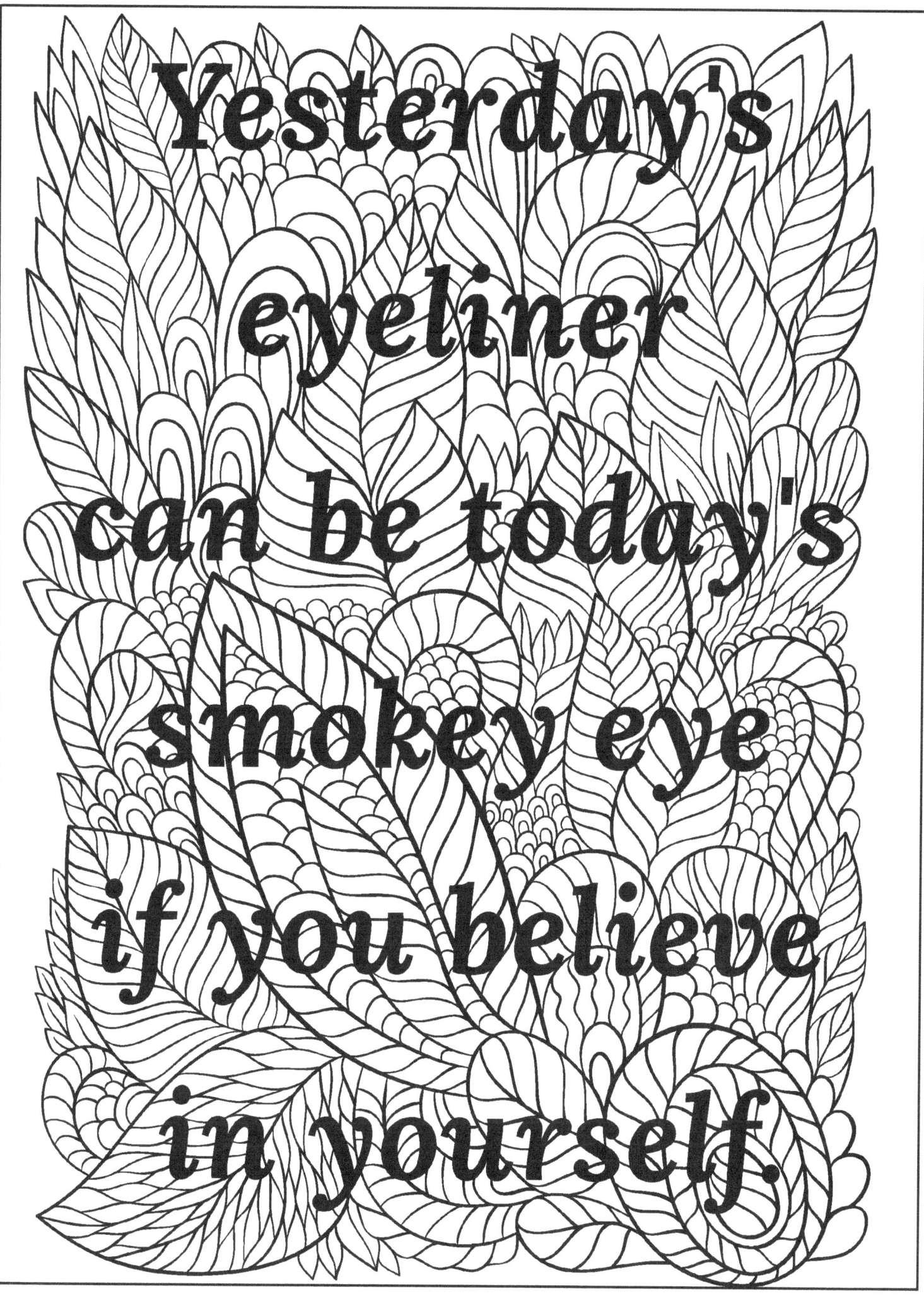

Yesterday's eyeliner can be today's smokey eye if you believe in yourself.

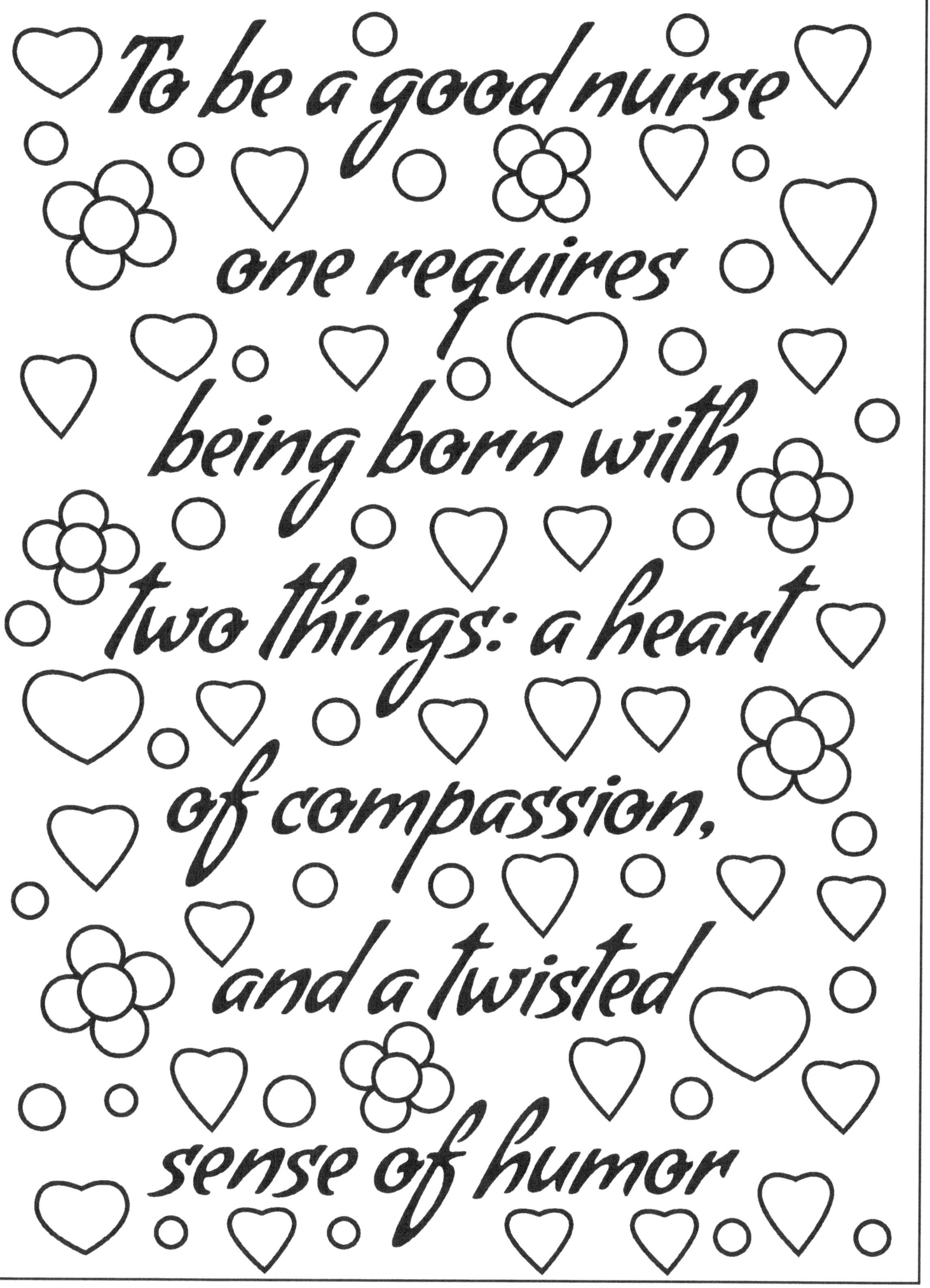

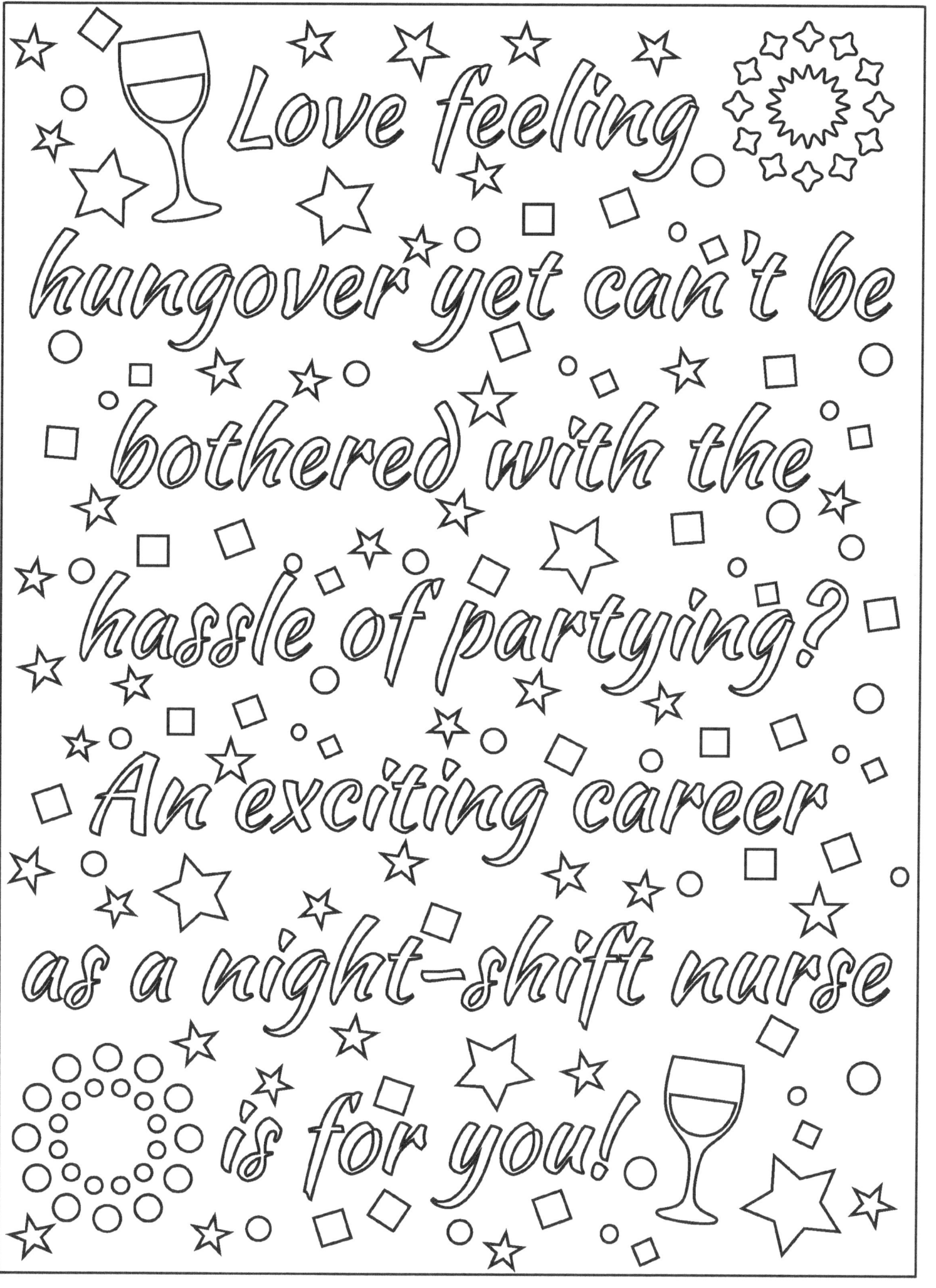

Love feeling hungover yet can't be bothered with the hassle of partying? An exciting career as a night-shift nurse is for you!

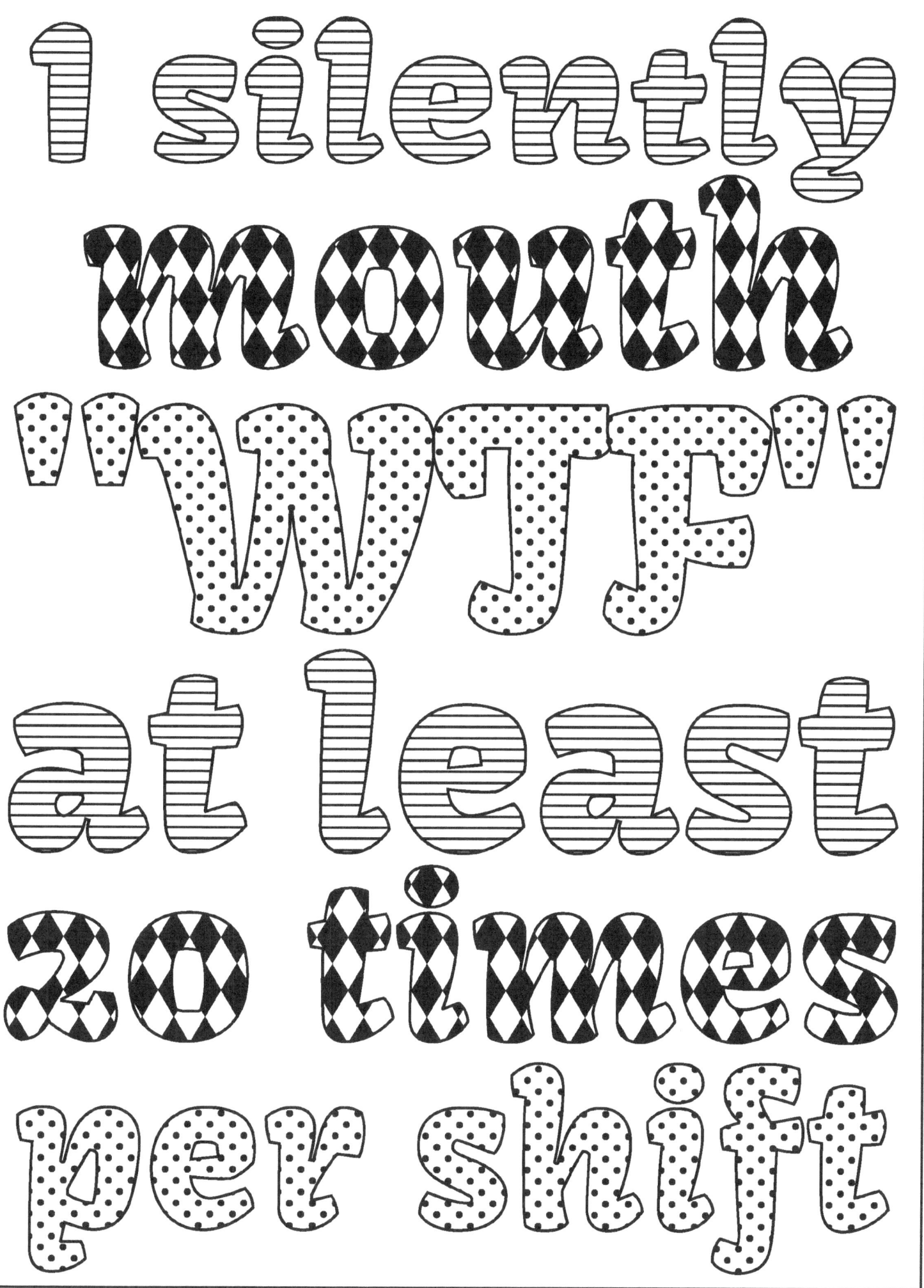

Nursing: A profession where you must also wash your hands BEFORE using the restroom.

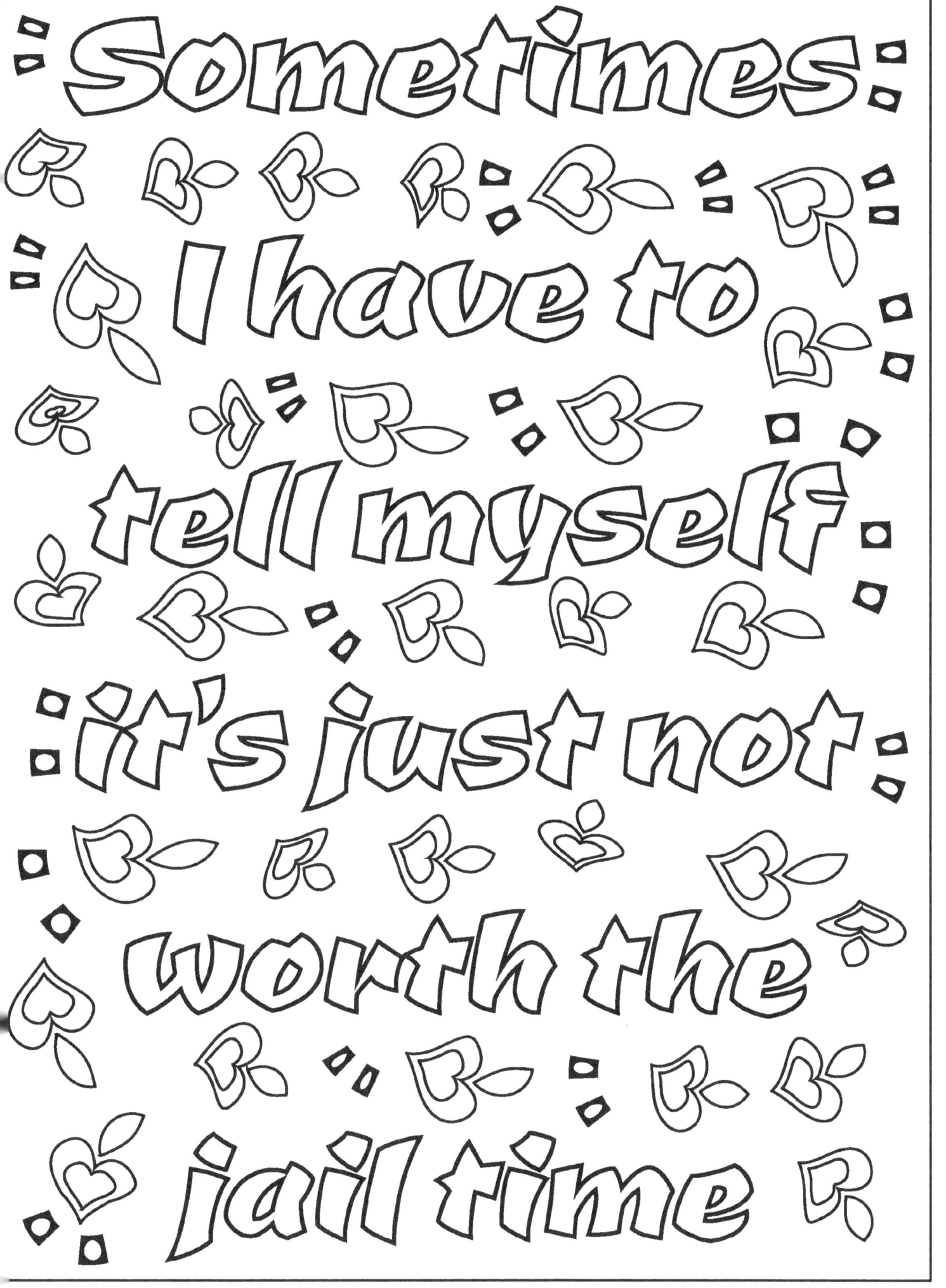

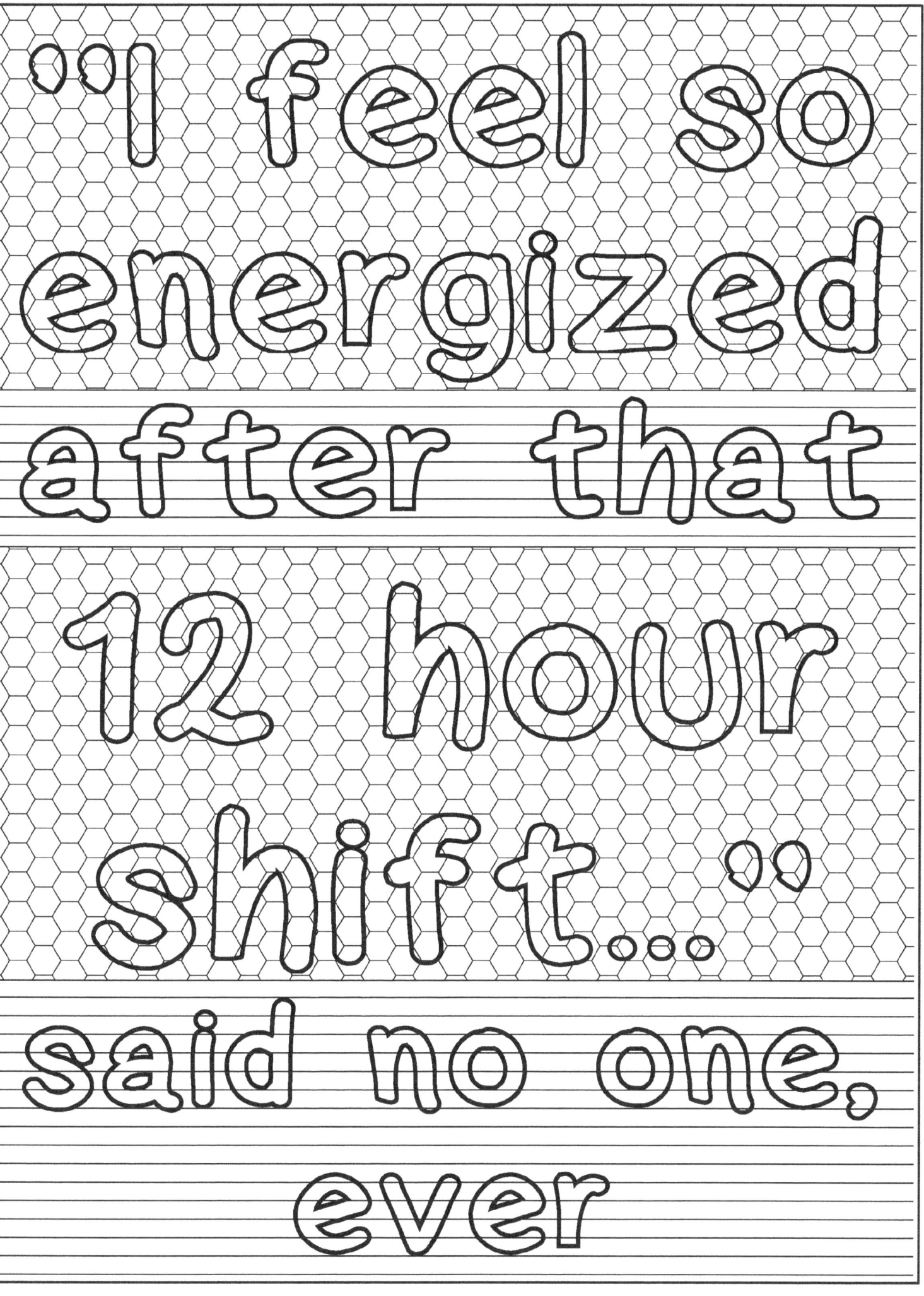

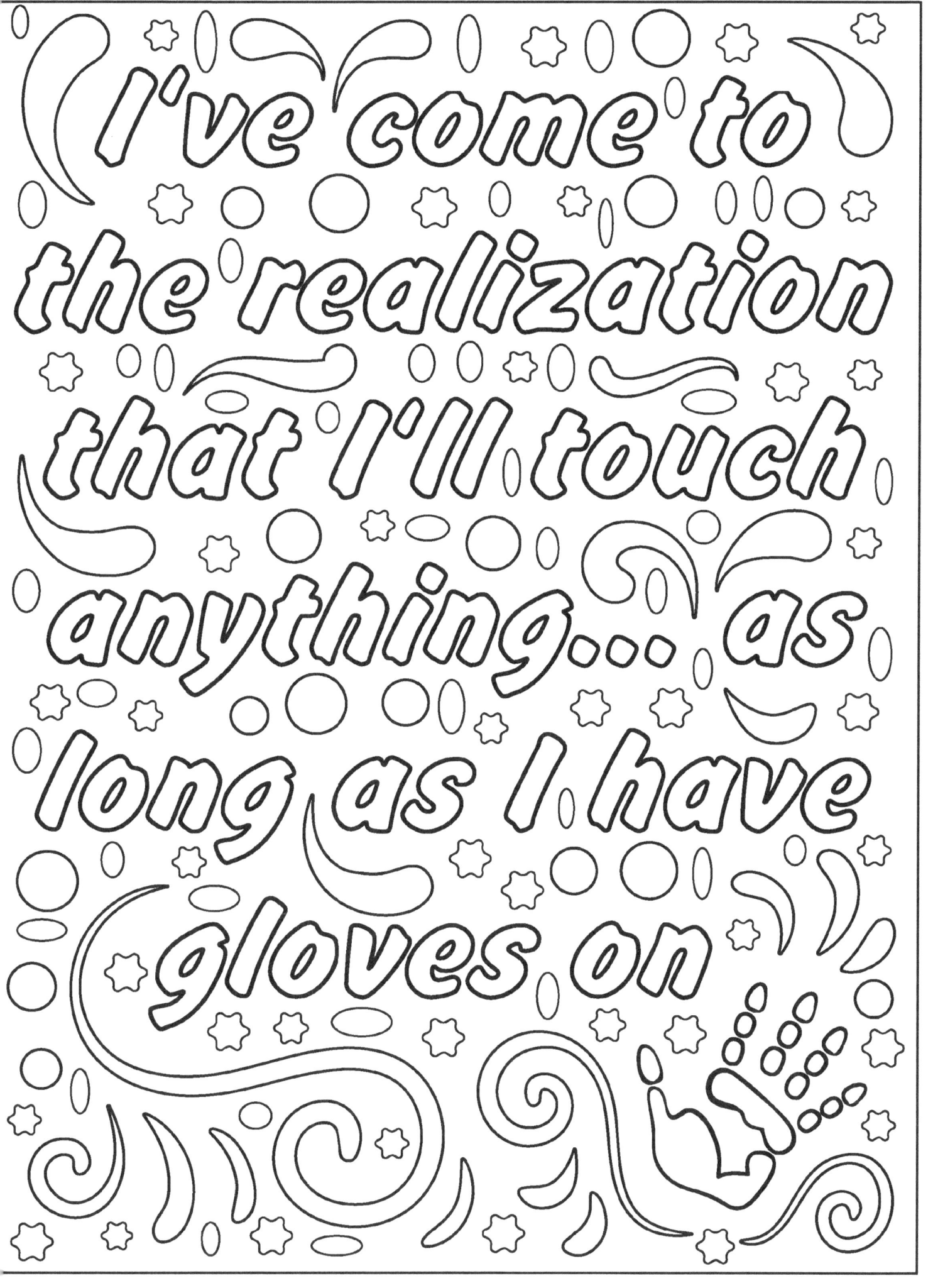

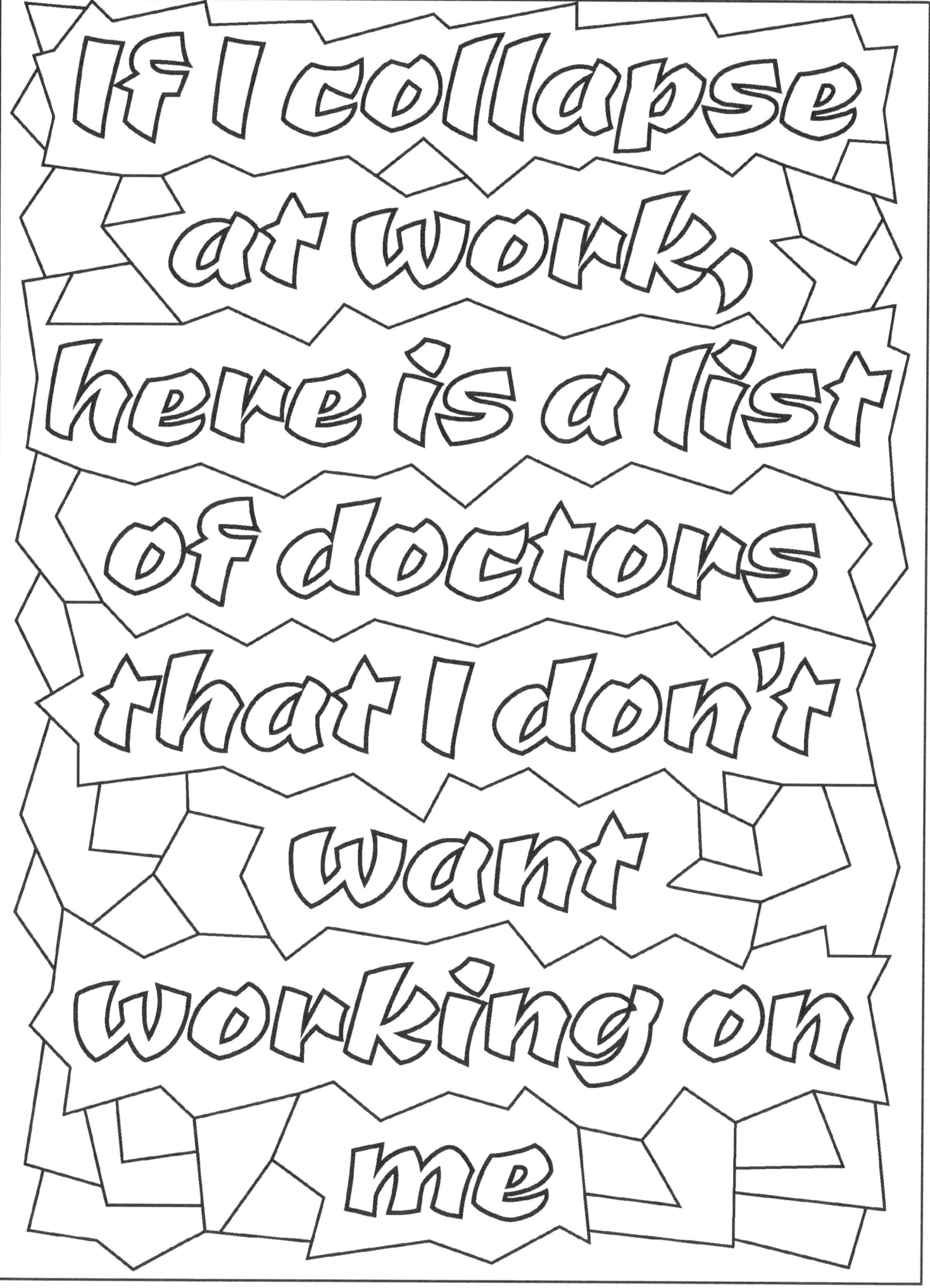

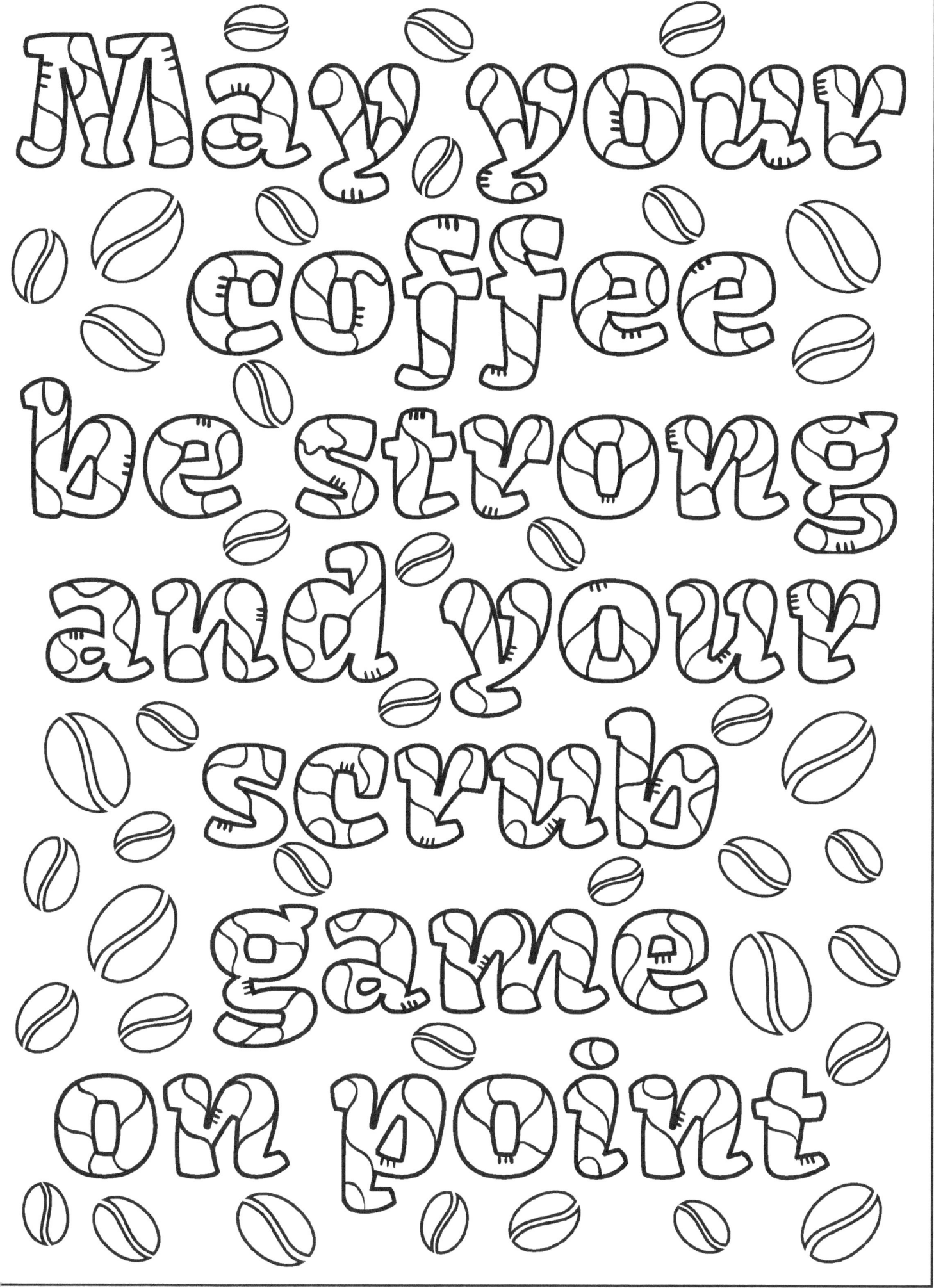

Sure I can do all your work while you sit there and do nothing all day. Why not I have nothing better to do!

NURSE

noun [en-juh-neer]
Someone who does
precision guesswork
based on unreliable
data provided by
those of questionable
knowledge.
See also:
wizard, magician

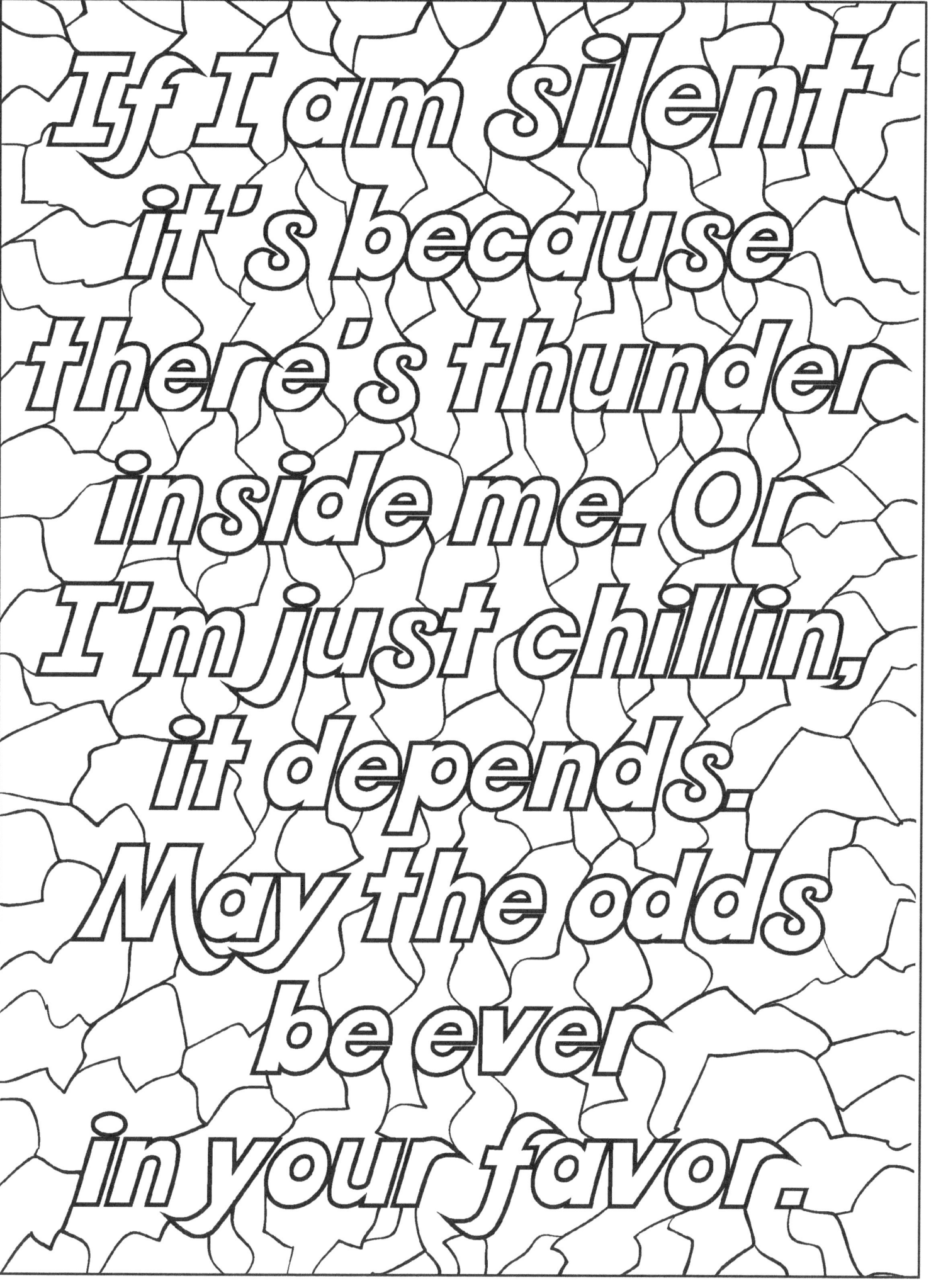

I'm sorry, putting up with your shit isn't on my to do list today.

You think Mondays are bad? Try working weekends, holidays, and 12 hour nights!

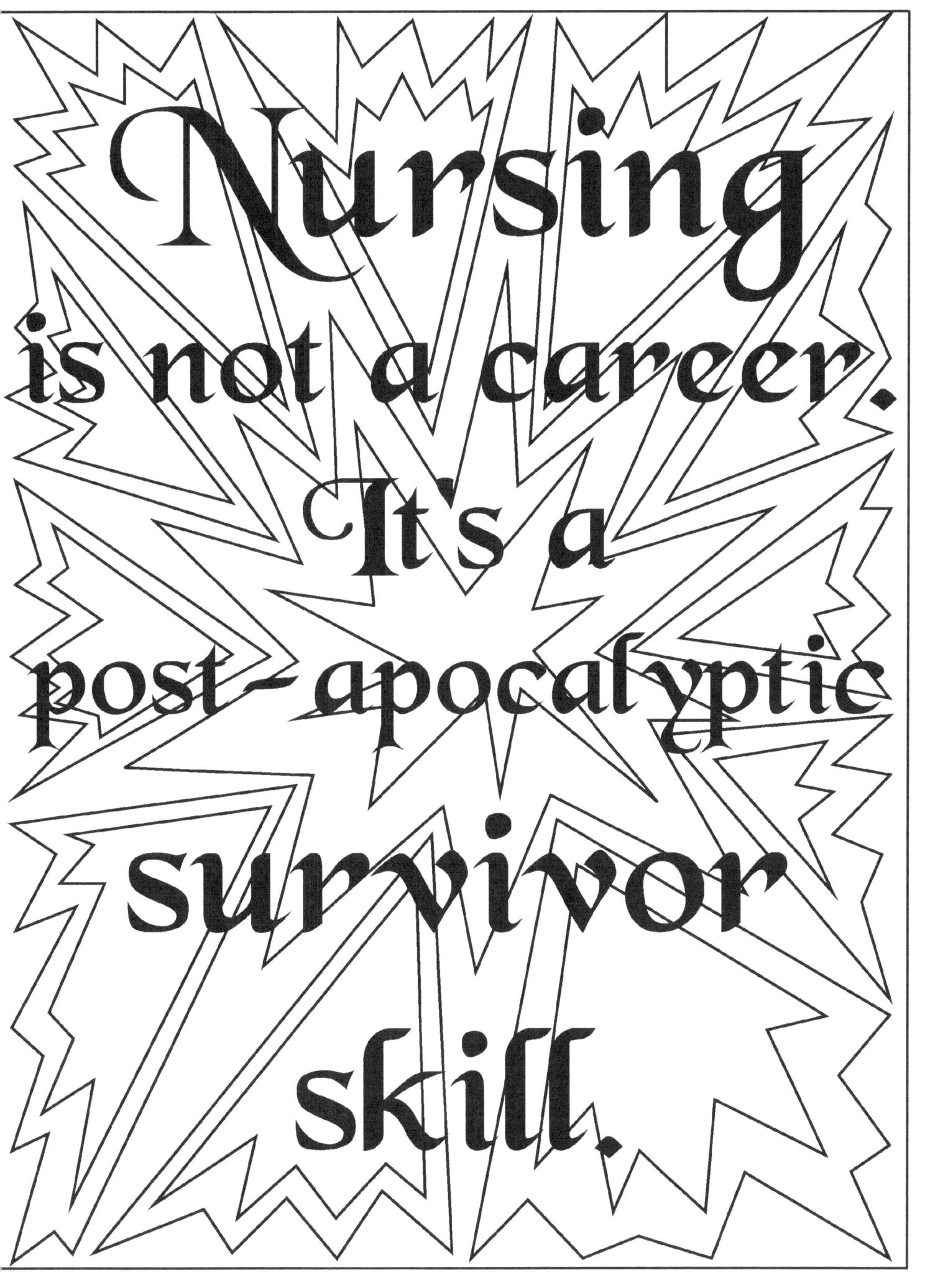

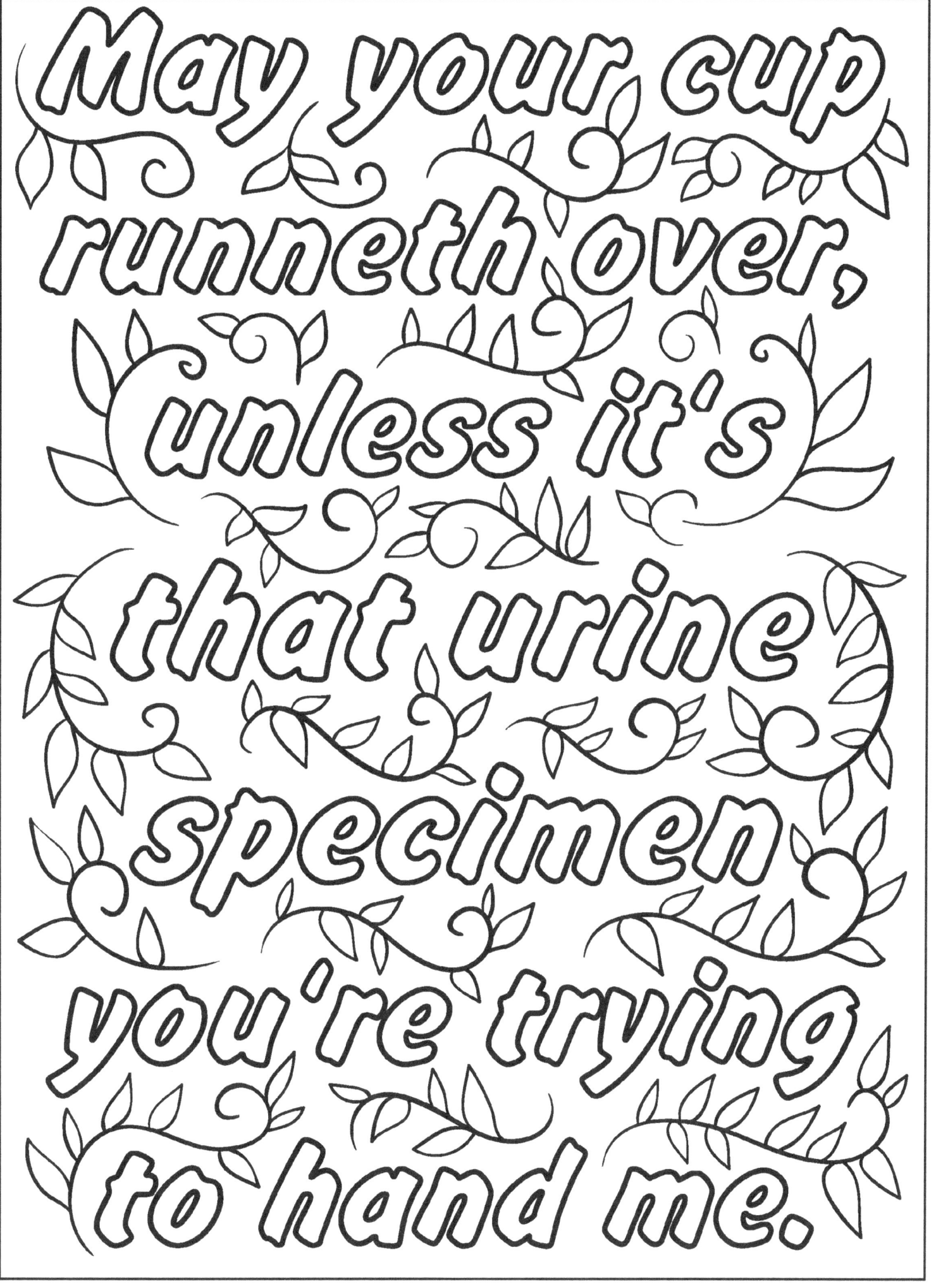

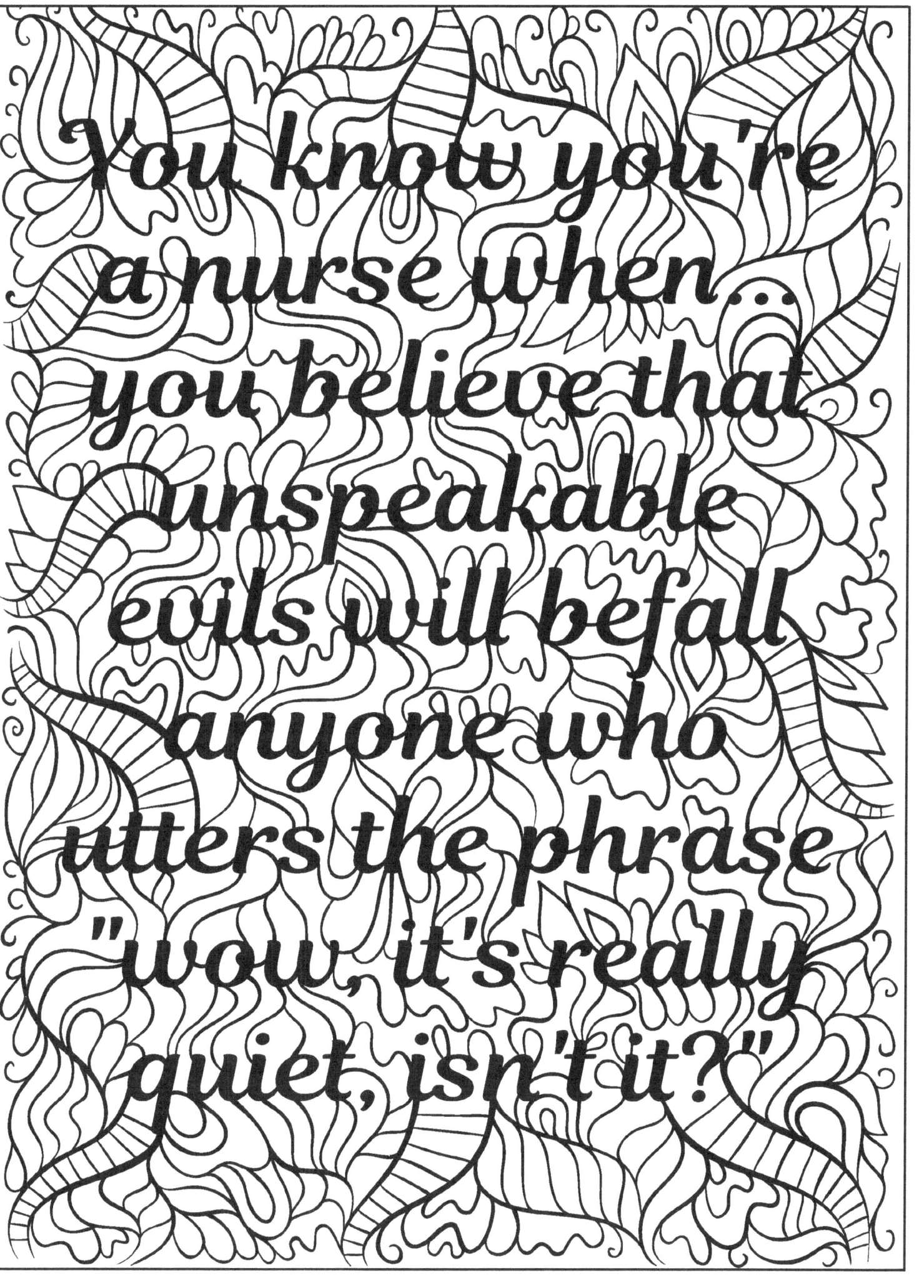

You know you're a nurse when... you believe that unspeakable evils will befall anyone who utters the phrase "wow, it's really quiet, isn't it?"

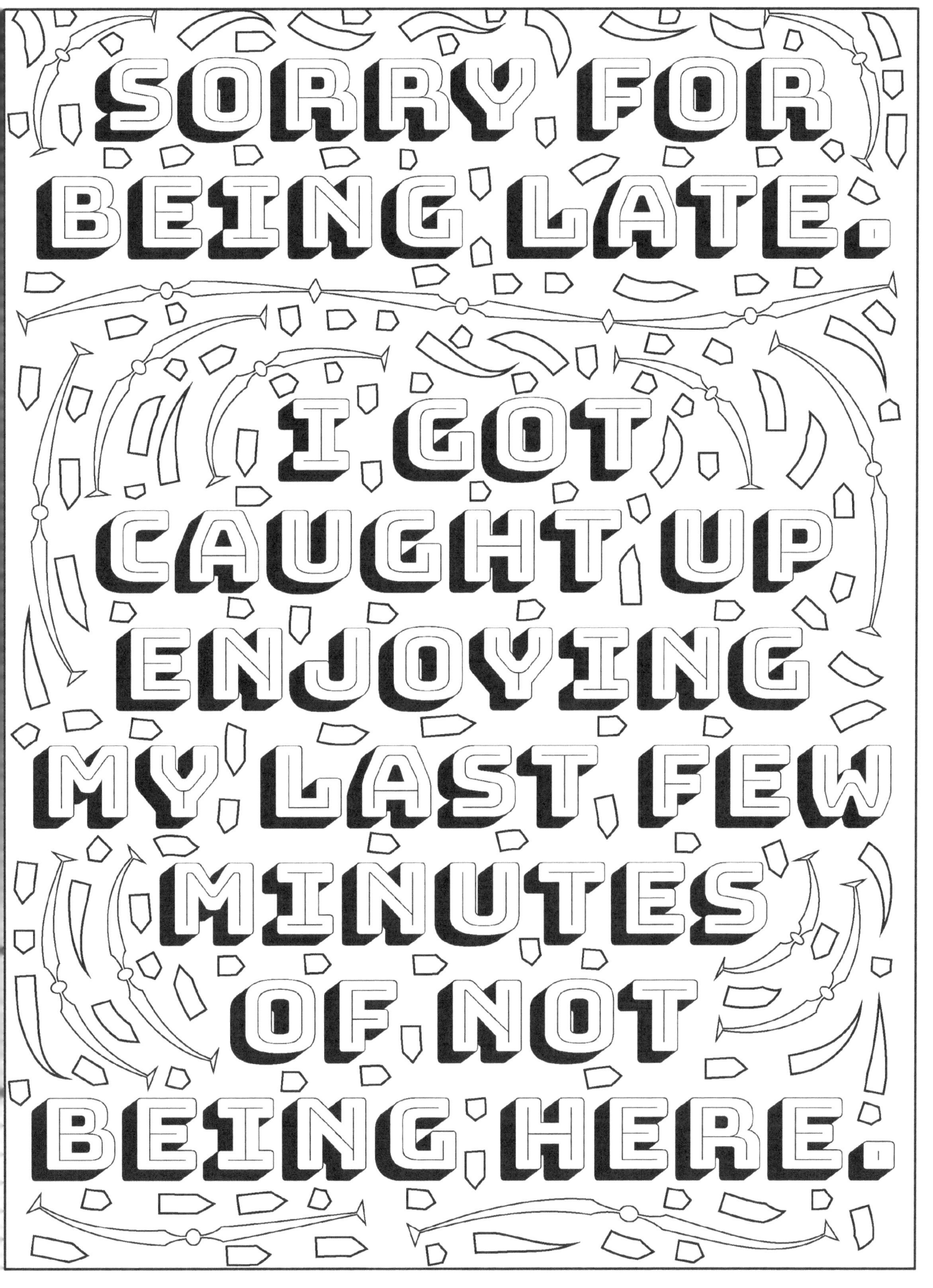

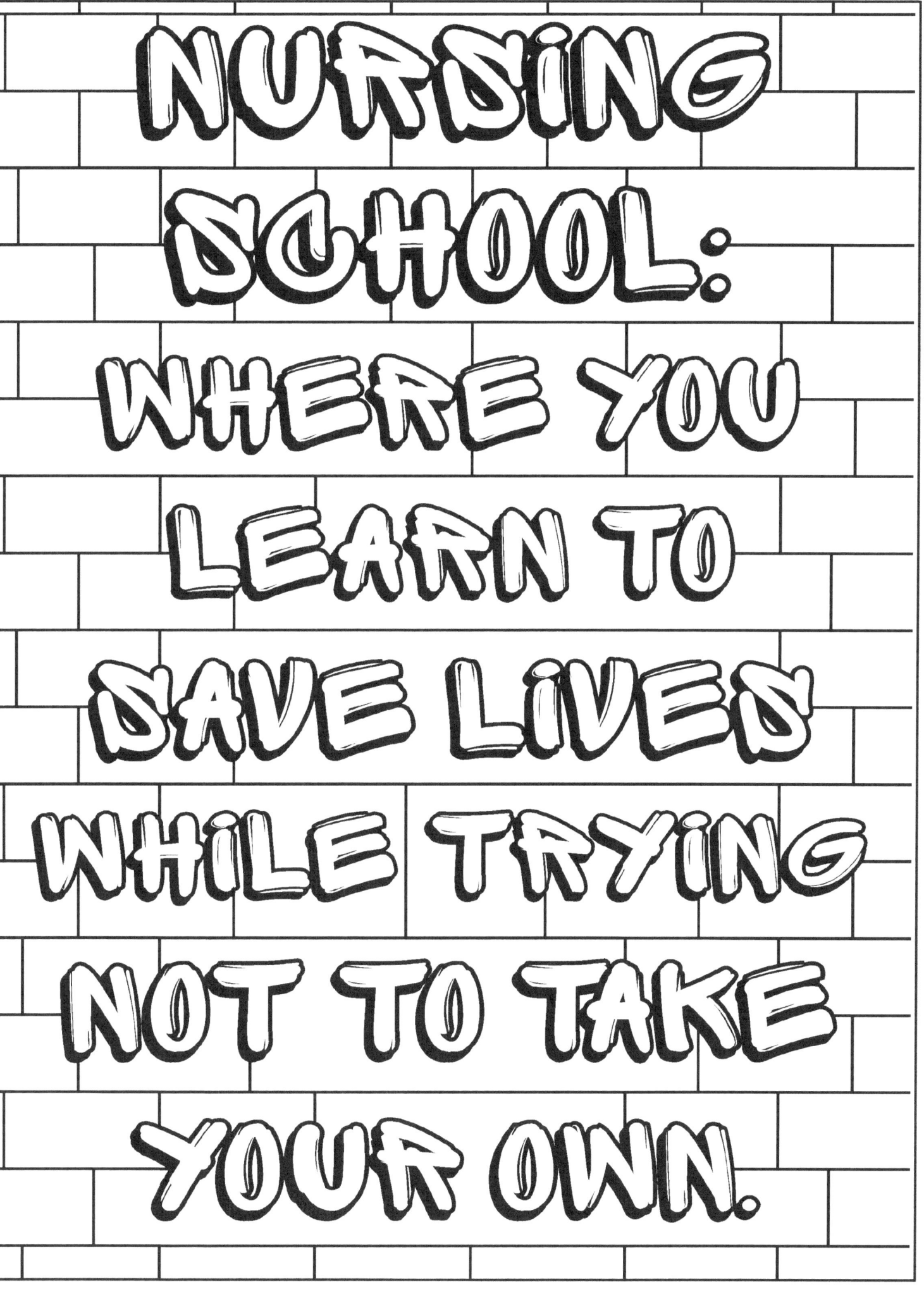

So you need a refill and you don't know what the drug is called? But it's white and round and you say???

They say you should walk a mile in someone else's shoes. I'm a nurse, and you'll be walking a hell of a lot further than that.

Please rate your pain on a zero to ten scale. Zero being no pain. Ten being I just force fed you live scorpions and then ripped off both your arms.

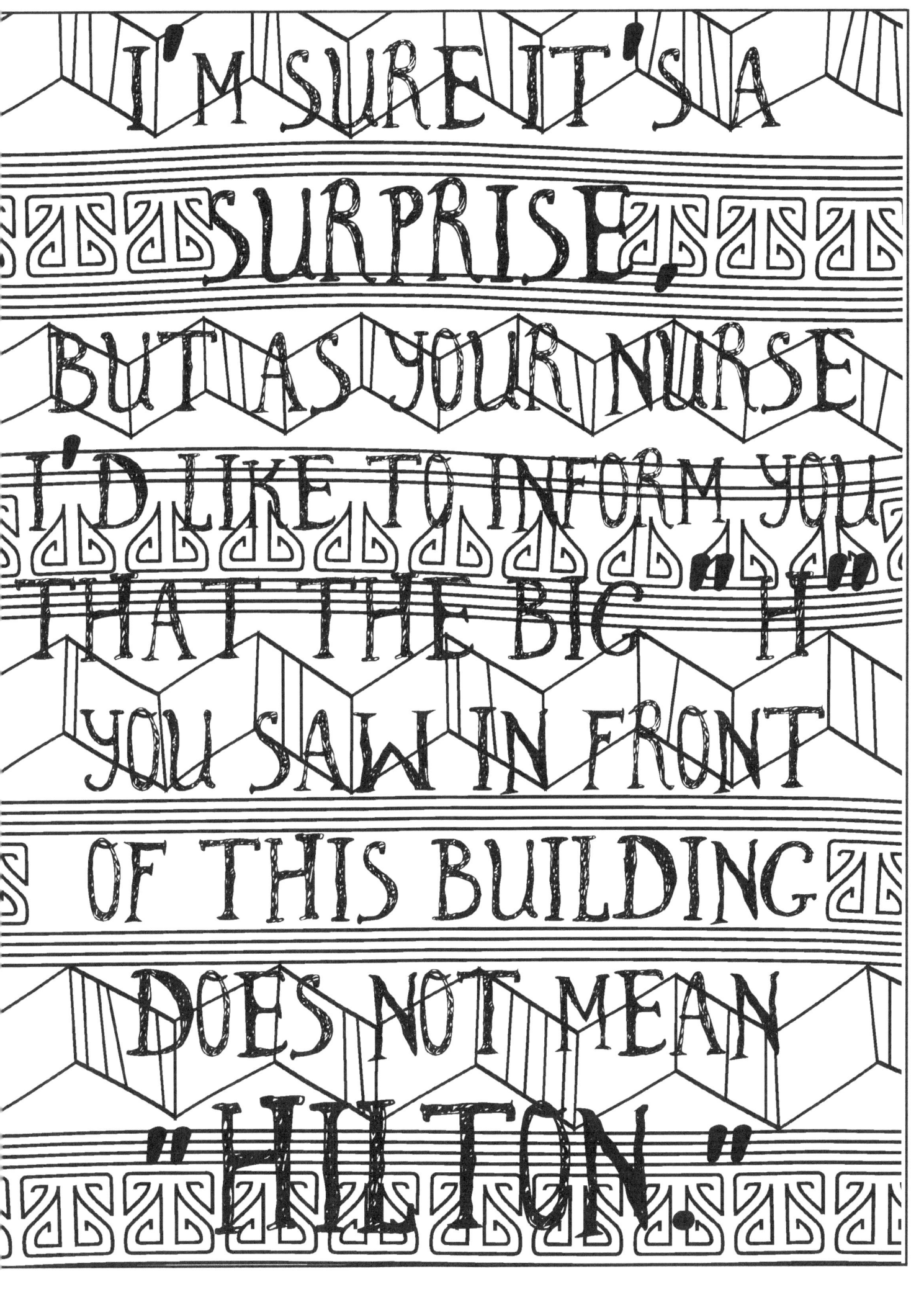

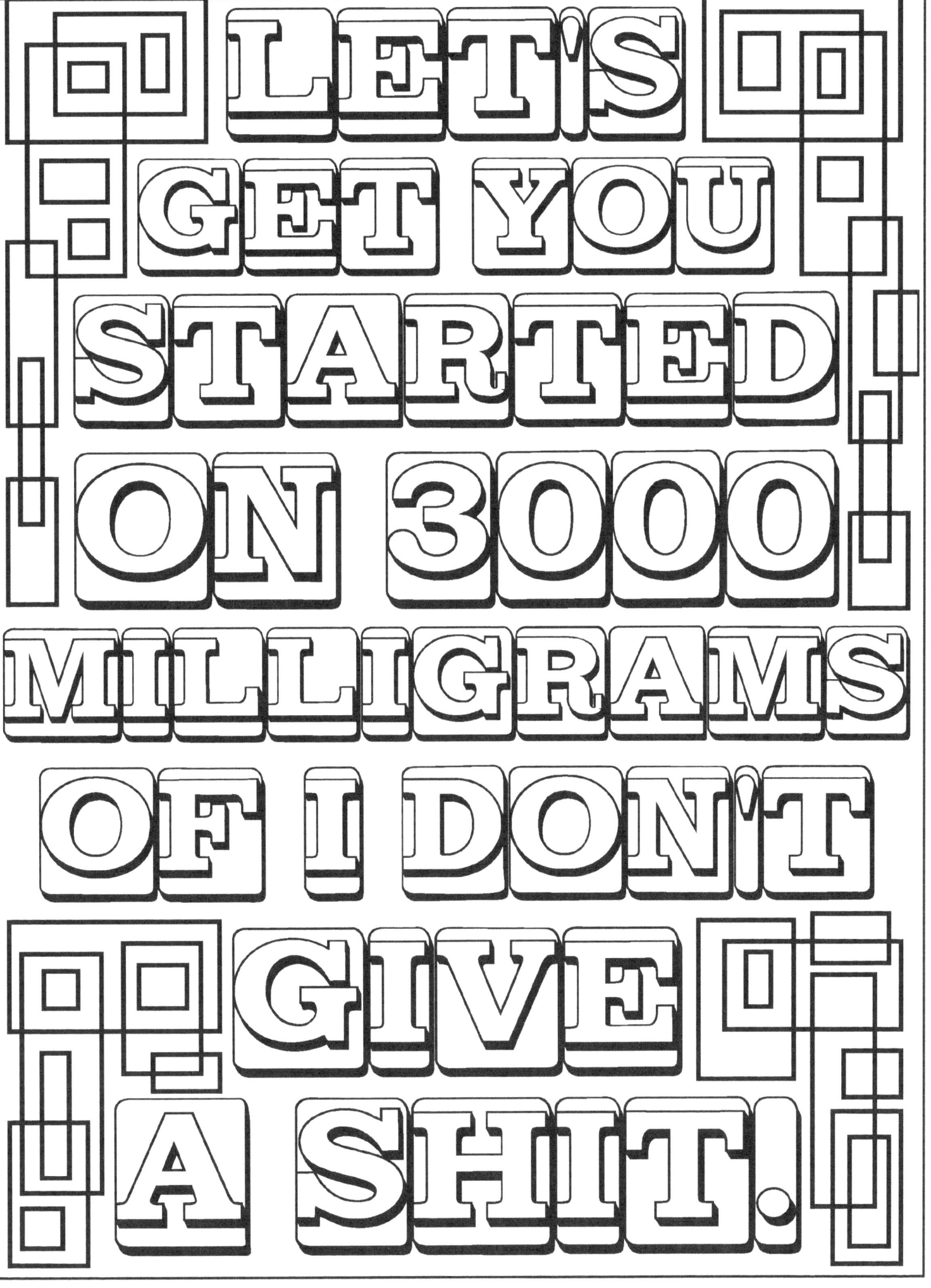

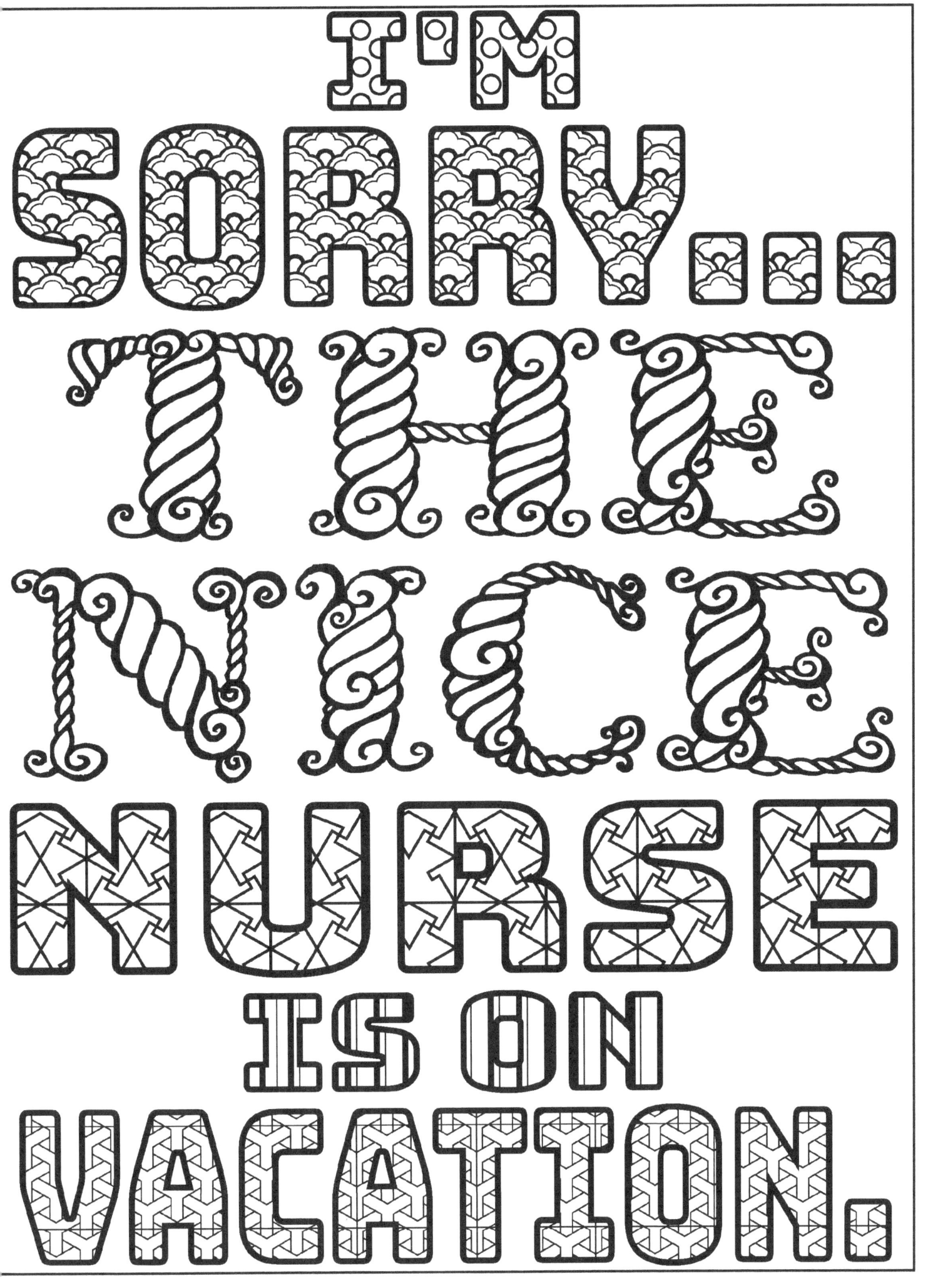

www.ingramcontent.com/pod-product-compliance
Lightning Source LLC
Chambersburg PA
CBHW081154180526

45170CB00006B/2075